"*Understanding Yoga Therapy* is an impressive, ̦ Marlysa Sullivan leads the reader through an intel philosophical roots and health benefits of yoga. W tion of physical postures and movements, but a system of movement deeper understanding of the human experience with the capacity to expand human potential."

— *Stephen W. Porges, PhD, Distinguished University Scientist, Indiana University; Professor of Psychiatry, University of North Carolina; and author of* The Pocket Guide to the Polyvagal Theory: The Transformative Power of Feeling Safe

"It is rare indeed to find a book that seamlessly blends the science, philosophy, and spirituality of yoga in a reader-friendly manner. This book integrates the best of the healing wisdom of Eastern traditions with the empirical approach of modern medical science, enhancing our perception of health, healing, life, and beyond. An especially admirable quality is the way Marlysa Sullivan has interwoven relevant stories from Indian culture into various chapters, thus enabling us to somatically 'feel' the experiential aspects of yoga therapy. She is indeed one of the brightest minds in modern yoga therapy, and this work is a substantial contribution to the field, indispensable to anyone wishing for a comprehensive understanding of yoga's transformative nature."

— *Yogacharya Dr Ananda Balayogi Bhavanani, MBBS, MD (AM), DSc (Yoga), C-IAYT, director, CYTER of Sri Balaji Vidyapeeth*

"*Understanding Yoga Therapy* is about personal transformation. This unique book demonstrates how the ancient teachings of yoga can be used clinically to help alleviate suffering. Yoga therapy is a new field of study, and there are many misunderstandings about how it is similar to or different from professions such as physical therapy, occupational therapy, and even psychotherapy. Once you read this book, you will understand how yoga therapy is uniquely positioned to help each of us heal our deepest spiritual wounds, as well as create balance on our mental, emotional, and physical layers. Yoga therapy is person-centered and focuses on improving function and also creating well-being—this book clearly explains how it works."

— *Amy Wheeler, PhD, C-IAYT, president, International Association of Yoga Therapists, and founder, Optimal State Yoga Therapy*

"Marlysa Sullivan takes her readers through an engrossing journey in *Understanding Yoga Therapy*. The journey begins with the yoga texts—the Upanishads, the epics, and of course, Patanjali's Yoga Sutras. The concepts relevant to yoga therapy are explained in a way which makes them easy to understand and apply in daily life. Concepts essential to understanding yoga, such as dharma, the trigunas, the pancha koshas, and the kleshas, are explained with clarity, with well-designed diagrams and appropriate references. Marlysa Sullivan ties up these concepts with those drawn from contemporary neuroscience and psychology, giving readers clarity about the psychophysiology of happiness, the polyvagal theory, and how yoga helps to achieve holistic healing and well-being. This book is a must-read for all those in yoga, as the author blends ancient and contemporary concepts concisely and in a very readable way."

— *Shirley Telles, MBBS, PhD (Neurophysiology), DSc (Yoga), director, Patanjali Research Foundation*

"With this masterful text, Marlysa Sullivan has cemented her position as the premier scholarly author on the application of yoga as a therapy. Unlike other texts that have overlaid a range of yoga principles and practices onto a contemporary health-science framework, *Understanding Yoga Therapy* is strongly founded in the full yoga framework, upon which a number of health-science principles are layered. All the multifaceted aspects of the yoga darshan as a path to well-being are explored, and the interweaving of contemporary health-science is remarkably seamless and honors the rich yoga tradition. This well-referenced and thorough text should become an essential part of every yoga professional's library."

— *Leigh Blashki, C-IAYT, founder, Australian Institute of Yoga Therapy*

Understanding Yoga Therapy

Understanding Yoga Therapy offers a comprehensive and accessible perspective on yoga therapy as a complementary, integrative route to promoting whole-person well-being.

Readers will come away from the book understanding how the philosophy, texts, and teachings of yoga benefit a wide range of health conditions. The book is split into three helpful sections: Part I discusses foundational texts and their interpretations; Part II outlines the biopsychosocial-spiritual and neurophysiological model of integrative health pertinent to yoga therapy; and Part III focuses on practical applications separate from the more familiar diagnosis-driven models. Experiential activities and case studies throughout the text illuminate how yogic practices can be incorporated for optimal health.

Bridging the ancient and modern, philosophical and scientific, *Understanding Yoga Therapy* offers a clear explanatory framework for yoga therapists, physicians, allied and complementary healthcare providers, and their patients and students.

Marlysa Sullivan is a physiotherapist, yoga therapist, and professor. Her research focuses on defining the framework and explanatory model for yoga therapy based on philosophical and neurophysiological perspectives.

Laurie C. Hyland Robertson is an editor and writer who specializes in yogic science and its intersections with healthcare. She is also a practicing yoga therapist.

Understanding Yoga Therapy

Applied Philosophy and Science for Health and Well-Being

**MARLYSA SULLIVAN WITH
LAURIE C. HYLAND ROBERTSON**

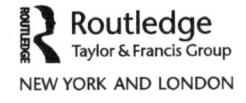

Routledge
Taylor & Francis Group
NEW YORK AND LONDON

First published 2020
by Routledge
52 Vanderbilt Avenue, New York, NY 10017

and by Routledge
2 Park Square, Milton Park, Abingdon, Oxon, OX14 4RN

Routledge is an imprint of the Taylor & Francis Group, an informa business

© 2020 Marlysa Sullivan and Laurie C. Hyland Robertson

The right of Marlysa Sullivan and Laurie C. Hyland Robertson to be identified as authors of this work has been asserted by them in accordance with sections 77 and 78 of the Copyright, Designs and Patents Act 1988.

All rights reserved. No part of this book may be reprinted or reproduced or utilised in any form or by any electronic, mechanical, or other means, now known or hereafter invented, including photocopying and recording, or in any information storage or retrieval system, without permission in writing from the publishers.

Trademark notice: Product or corporate names may be trademarks or registered trademarks, and are used only for identification and explanation without intent to infringe.

Library of Congress Cataloging-in-Publication Data
A catalog record for this title has been requested

ISBN: 978-1-138-48454-2 (hbk)
ISBN: 978-1-138-48455-9 (pbk)
ISBN: 978-0-429-50724-3 (ebk)

Typeset in Avenir and Dante
by Wearset Ltd, Boldon, Tyne and Wear
Printed and bound by CPI Group (UK) Ltd, Croydon, CR0 4YY

The practices in this book are in no way intended to be a substitute for consultation with a licensed healthcare professional. Please use them solely at your discretion and in conjunction with approved medical treatment. Neither the authors nor the publisher are responsible for any harm or damage caused by following any of the suggestions in this book.

Contents

About the Authors — *ix*
Acknowledgments — *xi*
Foreword by Richard Miller — *xiii*

Introduction — 1

PART I
Philosophical Foundations of Yoga as a Therapeutic Practice — 13

1 **The Path of Yoga** — 15

2 **Dharma, Ethics, and Right Action** — 30

3 **Foundations for Discernment: Understanding Prakriti, Purusha, and the Gunas** — 49

4 **Yoga Psychology: Body-Mind-Environment Relationships** — 68

5 **The Subtle Body: Exploring Tantra and Prana** — 86

PART II
Exploring Theoretical and Explanatory Frameworks for Yoga Therapy as an Integrative Healthcare Practice   111

  6 **Explanatory Model for Yoga Therapy to Promote Health and Well-Being**   113

  7 **Neurophysiological Perspectives**   132

  8 **From Conceptual to Practical Application: Biomedical and Yogic Perspectives on Yoga Therapy**   159

PART III
Applied Philosophy and Science for Health and Well-Being   181

  9 **Setting the Stage for Well-Being: Practices for Cultivating Sattva Guna and Regulating the Body-Mind**   183

10 **Cultivating Healthy Sensitivity: Interoceptive Skills and Discriminative Wisdom**   214

11 **Yogic Practices to Support Resilience and Transformation**   232

    Final Thoughts   254

    Index   *255*

About the Authors

Marlysa Sullivan, PT, C-IAYT

Marlysa is a physiotherapist and yoga therapist. She is an Assistant Professor in Yoga Therapy and Integrative Health Sciences at Maryland University of Integrative Health and holds an adjunct position at Emory University, where she teaches the integration of yoga and mindfulness into physical therapy practice in the Doctor of Physical Therapy program. She is the co-editor of *Yoga and Science in Pain Care: Treating the Person in Pain* as well as several peer-reviewed articles. Marlysa has been involved in the professionalization of the field of yoga therapy through the educational standards committee of the International Association of Yoga Therapists, which helped to define the competencies for the field, and in characterizing the yoga therapy workforce through research. Her research interests focus on defining the framework and explanatory model for yoga therapy based on philosophical and neurophysiological perspectives.

Laurie C. Hyland Robertson, MS, C-IAYT

After more than a decade in healthcare and business publishing, Laurie found her way to the transformative practices of yoga and then yoga therapy. She is now editor in chief of *Yoga Therapy Today* and managing editor of the *International Journal of Yoga Therapy* and contributes editorial services to a variety of yoga and wellness publications. Laurie divides her time between the extremes of a Costa Rican rain forest and the Baltimore-Washington area, where she owns Whole Yoga & Pilates.

Acknowledgments

This book represents an evolution of teachings, conversations, clinical work, and personal experience. I offer deep gratitude to the many students, clients, and friends who have been part of this process of learning and discovery.

I express immense gratitude to my husband, John Sullivan, who supports me in all the twists and turns of my career and interests, encouraging me to believe in myself and to follow my path. Thank you for being an inspiring partner in life and for always listening and being excited about discussing philosophy, spirituality, and science.

To the many friends, teachers, and family who have been amazing sources of support in my life I am immeasurably thankful: Carrie and Mark Anderson, Meredith Sullivan, Frances Shapiro, Tracey Meyers Sondik, Amy Wheeler, Corbett Oldham, Veronica Lewinger, Matthew Taylor, Leigh Blashki, Karen Davis Warren, Gordon Cummings, Leslie Taylor, Shelly Prosko, Neil Pearson, Diane Finlayson, Steffany Moonaz, Laura Schmalzl, Matt Erb, Madoka Chase Onizuka, Kelli Bethel, Tina Paul, Julia Romano, Kellie Finn, Ann Swanson, Erin Byron, Sherry Brourman, Melinda Atkins, Stephanie Lopez, and many others.

I would also like to express my sincere appreciation to those who helped me in the creation and writing of this book: Laurie Hyland Robertson for helping me find my voice as an author and for being able to bring the vision of this book to life in such a clear, strong, and creative way; Tzipporah Gerson-Miller for modeling the yoga postures, Anmarie Smith at DV Photo Video for the beautiful photographs, and Kristen Mercado for the space in which to take them; Catherine Behrent for your understanding and hospitality in having me as a guest as I wrote; Holle Black for your friendship and inspiring artwork; and to Routledge and Anna Moore for supporting this work and to Erin Byron for initiating this partnership.

My understanding of the material presented in Chapter 7 has been immeasurably deepened by work with respected colleagues including Matt Erb, Stephen Porges, Steffany Moonaz, and Laura Schmalzl.

Finally, my deep appreciation goes to Julie Wilcox for introducing me to the transformative healing capacity of yoga and for the encouragement to integrate this work into clinical practice; to Richard Miller, who has deepened my understanding of this work and supports my curiosity; and to Stephen Porges for being open to collaboration on a paper on polyvagal theory and yoga therapy and whose kindness and open-heartedness has served as a model of inspiration.

—Marlysa Sullivan

I am grateful to Marlysa for letting me ride along on this journey, share my thoughts, and shape her words. Heartfelt thanks to all of my teachers, and to my family and friends for always understanding when "I am working this weekend." And, most especially, eternal gratitude to Tom Hyland Robertson for sharing this life and supporting me in so very many ways.

—Laurie Hyland Robertson

Foreword

The sage Patañjali, in his ancient treatise on yoga, offers us the ultimate cure for ending suffering, be it our own or that of those who come to us as yoga therapists for healing. In his Yoga Sūtras, he addresses four fundamental questions that all healing modalities, including yoga therapy, need to resolve.

1. What is our condition *(heya)*?
   We are suffering, in dissatisfaction, pain, and confusion.
2. How did we get here *(heya hetu)*?
   The root cause of dissatisfaction is misperception or ignorance.
3. What is our goal *(hāna)*?
   The cessation of suffering through right understanding and action.
4. How do we arrive at our goal *(hānopāya)*?
   Through the path and means of yoga we can end our suffering by learning to discriminate between what changes *(prakṛti)* and what doesn't change *(puruṣa)*.

Patañjali understands that our human condition is dire. We are all ill. We are all suffering, even when we think we are not. Our body and mind are under constant attack by misperceptions, old age, sickness, and death. We are vulnerable to the onslaughts of our desires, anxieties, and fears; our social, interpersonal, economic, and political conflicts; and suffering that occurs as a result of our reaction to natural calamities around us such as accidents, fire, drought, famine, and climate change.

He understands that we are all seeking health and happiness. That we are interested in finding a means that can bring about a permanent end to our mental and physical suffering. To this end, Patañjali asserts that suffering can be cured. That if we are determined, we can bring an end to our suffering and attain our full human potential. And he points us to the means for ending suffering—an ultimate cure—a way of living that brings us to true health and happiness.

So what is health? What is illness? In the modern medical model health is the desired outcome, with illness labeled as abnormal. But our human bodies will never be perfectly free of disease, for illness and health are constantly in a battle for supremacy. What we call "health" entails only brief periods of homeostasis. And while we may be able to attain moments of homeostasis, we will all undergo death, and many of us illness and old age as well. Everlasting physical health is therefore only an illusion.

From the perspective of yoga therapy, true health and healing entail understanding that within us is an innate wholeness that can never be hurt or harmed and is never in need of healing. We are something vaster than our physical and psychological health. We possess a fundamental wholeness and well-being that is indestructible. For yoga therapy, curing the body and mind is not the ultimate goal, although it does offer interventions for restoring and maintaining physical and psychological health and well-being. But, more significantly, yoga therapy supports us to embrace a path that entails recognition of our innate wholeness, which is always healthy, no matter our state of body and mind.

We can never fully eliminate physical and mental anxiety and disease. But we can reduce the suffering we experience as a result of our misperceptions, ignorances, and ill-advised behaviors. Even when our body cannot be fully healed, we can still experience an inner sense of wholeness and health. Even as old age, sickness, and death arise.

Broadening our understanding of the healing that yoga therapy offers can deepen our appreciation of who and what we truly are. If we are only our body, and the thoughts, emotions, and experiences that we associate with it, then we will always desire to preserve the body at all costs. Under these circumstances physical health and healing will remain our most primary desire. But yoga therapy asks us to inquire into a deeper question: Are we more than our body, mind, and senses? Are we, perhaps, something that is luminous, unchanging, ever-present, and indestructible?

At its heart, yoga therapy is the application of yogic principles that empower us to realize our inherent wholeness and freedom from suffering. It invites us to awaken to our underlying essential nature that enables us to feel in harmony with ourselves, others, and the world around us, no matter our circumstance. It offers us educational processes that are designed to enhance health and wellness at all levels of our physical, psychological, and spiritual life. And it is comprised of non-dogmatic, secular approaches that respect our age, culture, religious and philosophical orientation, occupation, and mental and physical health. It teaches us how to live in the world, amidst our everyday conditions. It does not entail abstract teachings. It entreats us to come to firsthand knowing so that we bring these ancient teachings into the immediacy of our modern worldly life.

So it is my great pleasure that you now hold in your hands Marlysa's offering describing how to bring the depth teachings of yoga into your life, and into the healthcare system of our modern world. As she deftly points out, the yoga therapist is one who helps unpeel the layers that obscure recognition of our underlying wholeness, which leads to true health, equanimity, and steadfast joy and contentment. Here, the yoga therapist and client walk this journey together, for the yoga therapist is like a midwife who enables the student-client-patient to uncover and recover what has always been present. Marlysa offers us a salutogenic model that explores optimal states of health and well-being, echoing Patañjali's understanding that removing physical and mental disease is not enough. True health and healing are more than the absence of disease. They are the recognition of our true state of health, which is unbreakable and ever-present: innate wholeness of indestructible well-being.

Yoga therapy is therefore not just a science. It is an art that entreats us to be in tune with ourselves, our relationships, and the world around us. Marlysa offers us a book rich with philosophical insights and practical meditations and case studies that showcase how each concept offered can be utilized in the application of yoga therapy, within ourselves, and with the students-clients-patients we serve.

Understanding Yoga Therapy is a masterful guidebook that eloquently shows us how to recognize and embody our essential wholeness. Both profound and practical, this seminal work reveals the road we all must travel to embody our potential as fully alive and authentic human beings.

Richard Miller, PhD, co-founder, International Association of Yoga Therapists, and author, iRest Meditation: Restorative Practices for Health, Resiliency, and Well-Being

Introduction

How This Book Came to Be

Spirituality and its intersection with healing practices have been lifelong interests. These topics have influenced my path as a yoga practitioner and my perspective as a physical therapist seeking to apply a holistic perspective to health and well-being.

Some of my first college courses were in medical anthropology, where the topics included exploration of connections among spirituality, beliefs, medicine, and health. During this time, I also practiced and studied yoga with an interest in learning a holistic approach to healing. I had the good fortune to meet physical therapists, including Karen Davis Warren, Leslie Taylor, Gordon Cummings, and Matthew Taylor, who shared an integrative perspective. These teachers both mentored and supported me in entering the field while maintaining this holistic approach to client care.

With my knowledge of the body strengthened by training as a physical therapist, I still wanted to more deeply integrate a biopsychosocial-spiritual perspective into my work with clients. I pursued learning about the aspects of yoga that focused on philosophy and the more subtle aspects of the mind, energy, and spirit. Julie Wilcox and Richard Miller, along with training with the iRest Institute, have been the strongest influences in helping me to understand yoga's philosophy and subtle practices and apply them to my life and work.

I was fortunate to serve on the original Educational Standards Committee for the International Association of Yoga Therapists, which helped create competencies for yoga therapy schools. I also became involved in the first Master of Science degree program for yoga therapy in the United States at Maryland University of Integrative Health (MUIH). I created many of the courses and helped develop the clinic practicum, and I continue to teach in this program. The community of integrative health scholars at MUIH has supported my learning around research and the ability to bridge biomedical and philosophical thought with yoga therapy for healthcare and research contexts. I also had the good fortune to bring together an amazing group of colleagues, including Stephen Porges, Steffany Moonaz, Laura Schmalzl, Matt Erb, Kristine Weber, and Jessica Joy Noggle Taylor, to develop two papers clarifying an explanatory framework for yoga therapy and exploring the discipline's convergence with polyvagal theory for regulation and resilience.[1] Being part of the Global Consortium on Yoga Therapy has further connected me with visionary leaders in the field. Over the past 5 years, I have also taught an elective on the integration of yoga into physical therapy practice in Emory University's Doctor of Physical Therapy program.

All of these experiences have inspired this work on yoga therapy as a distinct and valuable practice and have informed the content of this book. However, integrating this knowledge into client care is what has helped me to understand the transformative power of yoga therapy. Working for over 15 years specializing in this integration of yoga therapy and physical therapy with chronic conditions has shown me the power of a truly biopsychosocial-spiritual approach to healing and well-being. Yoga therapy has provided me with the confidence and tools to have important discussions with clients on the relationships among belief, spirituality, emotion, and the body in a way that is accessible and meaningful to each person. In this book, my intention is to share the philosophy and applications to support readers in their own explorations of yoga therapy.

Yoga Therapy as a Distinct Complementary and Integrative Healthcare Practice

The rich and ancient wisdom tradition of yoga provides the context for yoga therapy. The practice must be completely grounded in this foundation to retain its full potential for improving well-being and to be understood as a distinct integrative healthcare profession. When yoga practices are taken outside this framework and applied through a solely biomedical lens, for instance, they may lose their effectiveness and therapeutic potential, creating possible misunderstandings of the practices themselves.

As an example, when a particular yoga posture is "prescribed" to correct a muscular imbalance for someone with low back pain, it might be a great practice but the prescription does not address the underlying causes of pain according to the yoga therapy explanatory framework. This not only limits the possible result, but also diminishes the scope of the yoga therapy profession and, possibly more seriously, mimics other modalities like physical therapy, leading to greater confusion for all.

If, on the other hand, that same patient with low back pain is seen through a comprehensive yoga therapy lens, the full array of yoga therapy practices, including pranayama, meditation, and ethical and lifestyle principles, can be used to address the underlying causes of the patterns that perpetuate pain. Even more significantly from the patient's point of view, these practices would include the philosophical concepts of yoga to facilitate a self-directed journey along a path toward well-being—regardless of whether the pain "resolves."

The same could be said of employing a breathing or meditation practice to alleviate stress, anxiety, or depression. Although these are useful tools, when not placed within this inclusive framework they may have limited effect. Such circumscribed applications diminish yoga therapy's capacity to function as an integrative healthcare practice. Understanding the principal philosophies and concepts that inform yoga therapy enables the practices' use in client-centered healthcare for the facilitation of well-being.

This book thoroughly defines the explanatory framework of yoga therapy to facilitate the practices' use to their full potential—helping clients experience well-being and work with the underlying causes of suffering. This framework illustrates yoga therapy's unique perspective and points the way to its integration into modern healthcare contexts. Broad themes that inform yoga's diverse traditions and lineages are elucidated alongside other philosophies and scientific thought that both support understanding and illustrate applications to client care.

Yoga therapy is a practice at once historically informed and thoroughly modern. The profession embodies the breadth of scope and adaptability to remain grounded in its roots while incorporating other philosophical and scientific material. To create a useful shared language for healthcare contexts we can link key yoga therapy concepts to philosophical and neurophysiological ideas such as phenomenology, eudaimonic well-being, ethical inquiry, polyvagal theory, interoception, top-down and bottom-up regulation, and resilience. Importantly, this approach places the practices, and their applications, into a therapeutic context that is both established in the philosophy that informed its development over time and can be understood as a distinct rehabilitative therapy for a variety of populations.

On Sharing Yogic Philosophy

Yoga philosophy is vast, and this book is not meant to be a definitive exposition of it. Rather, it is an offering of my own studies and how I have used these teachings in my work as a physical therapist and yoga therapist. I am opening a window onto my own path of integrating yogic tools into a therapeutic context for whole-person care. Yogic philosophy has offered incredible insight for both my personal and my professional lives. I hope that sharing the gifts I have received from studying yoga may help others to contextualize and apply it for the promotion of well-being.

Creativity, critical thinking, deep reflection, and the direct experience of these concepts are key. In high school, we read the same Shakespeare play in both drama and English classes. Our drama teacher, Tim Habeger, asked us to bring the play to life by exploring the meaning of its ideas within the context of our own lives. Conversely, our English teacher told us that there was only one correct interpretation of Shakespeare's words, negating our many different hypotheses and speculations. This book is offered in the former spirit—as a catalyst for discussion and reflection so that this timeless wisdom supports our professional and personal lives today.

The text is inherently limited by where I am in my own studies of yoga, spirituality, and philosophy. There are doubtless many other philosophies and topics I could have included, as well as different ways of explaining those that are discussed. The concepts explored here are those that have been pivotal in my life and work. They represent ideas that I have studied deeply enough to integrate into both my therapeutic work with clients and my teaching to students of yoga therapy and physical therapy.

The philosophies, teachers, and texts (including the choice of translations) discussed in this book represent those that have resonated deeply with me and provided insight for therapeutic application. My studies have been most profoundly influenced by the Samkhya Karika, Upanishads, Mahabharata, and Bhagavad Gita, so these texts constitute the majority of the referenced material. I have included some of the teachings of the Yoga Sutras of Patanjali where they clarified my teaching and clinical work.

As I continue to explore yoga, I know my approach will change; even the way I articulate some of these concepts will shift. I am grateful to teachers and mentors who have supported me at this intersection: wanting to offer the knowledge I have at this point, while knowing that my understandings will continue to grow and change.

Mostly, I hope to inspire an interest in these teachings so that readers will continue to explore yoga therapy's philosophical foundations. I hope to demonstrate that we can stay rooted to the integrity of yoga's wisdom tradition while evolving the practices for today's healthcare contexts. Yoga therapy is most importantly a living tradition—an extended dialogue through time—bridging the modern and historical, the philosophical and scientific.

Texts That Inform This Book

As mentioned, this book draws on several key yogic texts, including the Upanishads, Mahabharata (and its Bhagavad Gita), Samkhya Karika, and Yoga Sutras. Story is a powerful medium for shifting us from a more logical, cognitively oriented mindset to one that stimulates creativity, personal interpretation, and inner reflection. Direct quotes from the translations that have been meaningful to me are included so that readers can experience them alongside my own thoughts and commentary. I hope that sharing the stories will provide an entryway for thought that both honors the teachings and inspires further study.

This book is organized around key concepts that underlie the explanatory framework of yoga therapy, and the yogic texts included further describe these concepts. Timelines and authorship of these texts are very much up for debate and discussion. For more detailed information I recommend *The Roots of Yoga* by James Mallinson and Mark Singleton.[2]

Upanishads

The Upanishads are a collection of teachings with common themes, including the encouragement of inner reflection for answers about the outer world, a unifying principle beneath the ever-changing flux of the phenomenal world, and the importance of practical experience rather than intellectualized knowledge for direct realization of truth.[3] In the introduction to the version referenced in this book, Eknath Easwaran says that the etymology of the word *upanishad* suggests "'sitting down near': that is, at the feet of an illumined teacher."[4] These texts often present discourse between a teacher and a student and are thought to be among the earliest yogic texts (begun around the 7th century BCE).[5]

Bhagavad Gita and Mahabharata

The Mahabharata is an epic tale combining history and mythology. Its stories describe some of the key philosophies from both yoga and samkhya. The

Bhagavad Gita, part of the Mahabharata, includes teachings around a yoga of action—full engagement in life—while embodying yogic ideals. The Mahabharata, which began as an orally performed work, is a compilation of stories that were added to over time. The Bhagavad Gita is thought to have been added later in the Mahabharata's history.

This book refers to several versions of this text, including *Mahabharata: The Greatest Spiritual Epic of All Time* by Krishna Dharma, *The Mahabharata* by John D. Smith, *The Mahabharata* by Kisari Mohan Ganguli, and *The Bhagavad-Gita: Krishna's Counsel in Time of War*, translated by Barbara Stoler Miller.

Samkhya Karika

The teachings of samkhya can be found within other texts such as the Upanishads and Bhagavad Gita, but the Samkhya Karika represents a comprehensive description of this philosophical system. Concepts from samkhya inform yoga and yoga therapy as well as their sister science of ayurveda. Samkhya teaches a methodology for the alleviation of suffering through the development of discriminative wisdom between the spirit (purusha) and material nature (prakriti).

This book refers to several versions of the Samkhya Karika, including *Samkhya Karika* by Richard Miller, *Classical Samkhya and Yoga: An Indian Metaphysics of Experience* by Mikel Burley, and *Samkhya Karika* by Brahmrishi Vishvatma Bawra.

Yoga Sutras of Patanjali

The Yoga Sutras outline a path for disrupting the patterns of thought and action that create suffering. The Yoga Sutras represent a practical framework through which to understand the mental states that perpetuate suffering. This work offers an eight-fold path of discipline leading to the alleviation of that suffering.

The version referenced in this book is *Yoga: Discipline of Freedom: The Yoga Sutra Attributed to Patanjali*, translated by Barbara Stoler Miller, unless otherwise noted.

How to Use This Book

The capacity to experience somatically—via the body—a "felt sense" of philosophical principles has been crucial to my personal and professional integration of this material. When I ask readers to "feel" certain concepts—trust, patience, contentment, essential nature—I often offer lists of possibilities to allow for open-ended exploration and to reinforce the idea that there is no incorrect way to experience sensation. Yoga, as a practical philosophy, is ideal for this exploration, as it aims to move beyond the cognitive/intellectual to the lived/felt experience.

Meditations and practices are provided throughout the book to support an understanding of the material in the body as well as the mind. Readers are invited to contemplate the meaning and symbolism of the stories and concepts as they relate to and benefit their own circumstances. I offer my own interpretations, and how I have worked with these ideas, to support readers in finding their personal embodiment of the material. This method of dissemination is meant to begin a dialogue that enables individuals to explore their own authentic truth within this philosophy and to continue to develop these ideas for therapeutic application, transformative change, and greater well-being.

The first cohort of yoga therapy students at MUIH created an acronym for my style of teaching this embodiment of concepts: DREME stands for Discover and Release of Emotional and Mental Energy. During these early classes, we would first have a discussion on a philosophical principle like contentment or essential nature. I would next lead an introspective, reflective yoga practice asking the students to discover what was arising in the bodily experience, to then work with what was needed to release tensions (be they physical, mental, emotional, or energetic), and finally to embody the concept itself. I would leave the actual choice of postures, breathing techniques, meditations, or visualizations up to the students—they generated them from the insights they garnered during this reflective process.

For example, we might begin with a statement like, "Yoga's ancient wisdom tradition helps us to explore the nature of suffering and a path for freedom from such suffering."

- I ask readers to reflect on what this means by asking questions: What is meant by "suffering," and what is meant by "freedom from such suffering"? The end of all unhappiness, unease, or pain? Or is freedom from suffering referring to something more subtle? And how do we apply this idea in a therapeutic yoga context?
- A meditation or inquiry then prompts discovery of how readers physically and mentally/emotionally experience these concepts—the "felt" experience:
    ○ Take a moment to consider the ideas of suffering and freedom from suffering. Notice the experience of these ideas in your body—where

might your attention be drawn, and what kinds of sensations are felt there (hardness/softness, fullness/emptiness...)? Is there a movement or body position that characterizes these concepts? Notice also what might arise in your mind as you hold these ideas of suffering and freedom from suffering—what other beliefs, thoughts, and emotions surface? Continue to notice what arises mentally and physically as you reflect and experience these concepts of suffering and freedom from suffering in your mind and body.
- Reflect on what you learned about how you relate to these concepts. How might you use the body position, movement, or sensation to strengthen the feeling of freedom from suffering? How might you use the emotions, thoughts, and beliefs that arise around freedom from suffering to create an affirmation for yourself?

These experiential practices, as well as clinical examples, are woven throughout the book, but Part III focuses particularly on the therapeutic applications of yogic tools. (Audio versions of the practices are available at understandingyogatherapy.com.) All of the clients described in the text are real, although their names and details about their circumstances have been changed to protect their privacy.

A Brief Outline

As you read this book, I invite you to be an active participant, to pause, explore, and reflect on concepts or sections that either resonate or don't resonate with you. Working with texts that offer experiential practices allows readers to pause and integrate the concepts. I have often enjoyed books that I worked with for months at a time and hope to have created that opportunity here.

The order of this book also represents a learning style that resonates with me: first diving into yogic and complementary philosophies, followed by the contemporary sciences that can inform the way we understand concepts, and concluding with clinical applications. Some readers may want to start with Part II for the scientific and integrative health perspectives; others may want to begin with the applications in Part III.

Part I, "Philosophical Foundations of Yoga as a Therapeutic Practice" (Chapters 1 to 5), focuses on the framework provided by yogic texts as well as teachings from Aristotle and Viktor Frankl. Essential nature, dharma, eudaimonia, virtue ethics and ethical inquiry, nature of the mind, gunas, koshas, tantra, and phenomenology are all explored in relation to yoga therapy's guiding principles.

Part II, "Exploring Theoretical and Explanatory Frameworks for Yoga Therapy as an Integrative Healthcare Practice" (Chapters 6 to 8), considers scientific parallels and convergences that provide a model and translatory language for yoga therapy's biopsychosocial-spiritual perspective. Topics include the science of eudaimonic well-being, spiritual and social well-being, polyvagal theory, systemic body-mind regulation, and resilience. Chapter 8 includes a discussion of the holistic application of yogic practices including yama/niyama, asana, pranayama, and meditation. Although there are other yogic tools, such as mudra and chanting, I have included these four because they are what I have most often used with clients.

Part III, "Applied Philosophy and Science for Health and Well-Being" (Chapters 9 to 11), focuses on application of the practices of yama/niyama, asana, pranayama, and meditation for body-mind regulation, interoception and discernment, and resilience. Chapter 9, which explores ways of promoting body-mind regulation, includes a number of experiential practices for readers and clients, along with tables illustrating example asana. Chapters 10 and 11, in particular, offer clinical examples of the inquiry practices offered to encourage discriminative wisdom and resilience. (Note that here and in all other instances client names and identifying details have been changed to protect individuals' privacy.)

Choices, Biases, and Terms

The Challenge of Providing Practices

When I first became a yoga teacher, I had difficulty answering students who would ask me what pose would help X condition. As a physical therapist, I could not answer their question because I would need to do a detailed assessment and work with them over time to understand their needs in the context of their life circumstances. Likewise, as someone interested in yoga therapy as a whole-person intervention, I would want to employ the full yogic framework to support them in a process of transformative change and improved well-being. A reductionist approach would only short-change what yoga could offer while providing, at best, short-term relief of their complaint.

This book does not offer prescriptive sequences or suggested poses "for" specific conditions. Rather, it lays out guidelines for yoga therapy based on a biopsychosocial-spiritual approach to supporting health and well-being. The applications chapters are divided into practices that may be beneficial to a variety of conditions and client populations as they support body-mind regulation, interoception and discriminative wisdom, and resilience. The poses and practices included are a "greatest hits" of sorts, representing those I use most often and have found most helpful for a wide range of clients. I do offer suggestions on why and how the practices might be used, but readers must be aware of the complexity of applying any one of them to any one uniquely nuanced, intricately developed human. Training as a yoga therapist ideally involves many hundreds or thousands of hours of direct study of unique beings and their patterns of stress and ease.

Many books complement this discussion and its application to clinical populations. Some of those I recommend and use often include *Yoga and Science in Pain Care: Treating the Person in Pain*; *Yoga Therapy for Arthritis*; *Yoga for Healthy Aging: A Guide to Lifelong Well-Being*; *Yoga as Medicine: The Yogic Prescription for Health and Healing*; and *Yoga for Emotional Balance*.[6]

Terminology

Yoga therapy has helped me develop a language and methodology to work with the subjective nature of pain, suffering, and well-being. "Subjective nature" here refers to the idea that the objective presence of difficulty, disease, illness, or pain does not always correlate with individuals' reports of stress, pain, or suffering. Yoga's framework includes a process of inquiry into how we interpret and relate and react to what is happening within the body, mind, and environment. In this terminology "body" includes all the structures and systems of the physical and energetic body; "mind" includes thoughts, emotions, beliefs, and habitual responses; and "environment" includes the individual's context, including life situations and circumstances. The term body-mind-environment or BME is used throughout the book to differentiate these "outer" experiences" from one's essential nature, which yoga aims to help us realize.

In writing this book, Laurie and I had many discussions about the use of gendered pronouns and the possible perpetuation of exclusionary language of all kinds. Although the source texts almost exclusively use male characters and masculine pronouns when describing knowledge-seekers, we chose to use *they* instead of *he/she* or *he or she* and to purposefully include more female pronouns where the individual form is appropriate.

Another choice we made was how we would use Sanskrit terms. We elected to use common phonetic spellings without diacritics. Much more could be said about this choice, too, but in the end we decided that it not only makes the material more accessible, but also supports our intention to facilitate the integration of yoga therapy into healthcare and research contexts.

This is an exciting time for integrative health and the evolution of yoga therapy as an accessible and widespread healthcare practice. Each time I have the opportunity to welcome another cohort of MUIH yoga therapy students, find out about what graduates are doing, or meet other yoga therapy professionals throughout the world I am inspired and encouraged by the possibilities to help others through this work. I am grateful for the opportunity to be a part of this profession and to offer this book. I hope it proves helpful in bringing yoga therapy to many communities for healing.

Notes

1. Sullivan, M. B., Erb, M., Schmalzl, L., Moonaz, S., Noggle Taylor, J., & Porges, S. W. (2018). Yoga therapy and polyvagal theory: The convergence of traditional wisdom and contemporary neuroscience for self-regulation and resilience. *Frontiers in Human Neuroscience, 12*(67); Sullivan, M. B., Moonaz, S., Weber, K., Taylor, J. N., & Schmalzl, L. (2018). Toward an explanatory framework for yoga therapy informed by philosophical and ethical perspectives. *Alternative Therapies in Health and Medicine, 24*, 38–47.
2. Mallinson, J., & Singleton, M. (2017). *Roots of yoga*. London: Penguin.
3. *The Upanishads* (Vol. 2), translated by Eknath Easwaran, founder of the Blue Mountain Center of Meditation, copyright 1987, 2007; reprinted by permission of Nilgiri Press, P. O. Box 256, Tomales, CA 94971, www.bmcm.org.
4. Easwaran, *The Upanishads*, p. 19.
5. Mallinson & Singleton, *Roots of yoga*.
6. Moonaz, S., & Byron, E. (2018). *Yoga therapy for arthritis: A whole-person approach to movement and lifestyle*. London: Singing Dragon; Bell, B., & Zolotow, N. (2017). *Yoga for healthy aging: A guide to lifelong well-being*. Boulder, CO: Shambhala Publications; McCall, T. (2007). *Yoga as medicine: The yogic prescription for health & healing: A yoga journal book*. New York: Bantam; Pearson, N., Prosko, S., & Sullivan, M. (2019). *Yoga and science in pain care: Treating the person in pain*. London: Singing Dragon; Forbes, B. (2011). *Yoga for emotional balance: Simple practices to help relieve anxiety and depression*. Boston, MA: Shambhala Publications.

Part I

Philosophical Foundations of Yoga as a Therapeutic Practice

The Path of Yoga   1

Background

The wisdom tradition of yoga represents a complex, evolving system intended to help us develop insight into the causes of suffering and its alleviation. The tradition includes both a rich philosophical foundation and specific practices that serve as a methodology for this exploration.

Often, yoga is thought of as a set of practices consisting of some combination of physical exercises *(asana)*, breathing techniques *(pranayama)*, and forms or stages of meditation. However, these practices are situated within a historical and philosophical context that must be understood for optimal application. Performing the practices without knowledge of their context, intention, or goal is akin to trying to find your way to a dinner party without knowing the location, or trying to cook a meal without knowing what dishes you were trying to cook. Recognizing that these practices are part of a comprehensive methodology is essential. Within this context, specific teachings can be placed along the way as markers to help practitioners on the path toward the alleviation of suffering.

Historically, yoga has been described as a state characterized by freedom from suffering and realization of our essential nature, as well as the practices that lead to that goal.[1] Yoga scholar, teacher, and creator of iRest yoga nidra meditation Richard Miller describes yoga as both the action of awakening to, and a description of, our underlying undivided essential nature.[2] Part I of this book explores yoga as this realization that enables us to mitigate suffering. The later sections of the book describe the methodology and practices that lead to this aim.

Philosophical Foundations of Yoga

The word yoga is sometimes defined as *unity*. This idea of union often includes some combination of body and mind or body, mind, and essential nature/spirit. Recognizing yoga as more than a set of practices—as an experience of unity to which the practices direct us for the alleviation of suffering—is essential to applying the philosophy and practices for therapeutic purposes. Understanding this overall intention also helps to clarify the many types of yoga being taught. Just as there are many paths up the mountain, many sets of practices can lead practitioners to this aim of yoga. Each individual must find for herself the practices that cultivate unity. The texts on which we draw offer diverse practices—with most including asana, pranayama, meditation, and *yama* and *niyama* (ethical principles for conscious living)—all applied to the goal of liberation from pain or suffering.

Yoga teachings offer insight into how practitioners can change their reactions and relationships to body, mind, and environmental phenomena in pursuit of unity. This process empowers us to notice and change habitual reactions that perpetuate suffering. The practices elucidate ways of interacting with body, mind, and life that ease or even resolve suffering. Yogic philosophy is practical and intended to be both contemplated and applied to everyday life.

Teaching Through Story

Oral traditions were the primary method of disseminating ideas before writing became the dominant form of communication. The use of story provides an ideal format for teaching the nuances of yogic wisdom. Both story and metaphor enable sharing of complex ideas through symbolism. Listeners are then able to determine personal meaning and application to their own circumstances. As symbols and story can be interpreted in a multitude of ways, they offer a means of sharing essential teachings across time and cultures.

Yoga therapy has this rich yogic tradition as its foundation, underpinning a distinct and unique perspective. Understanding the intentions behind the stories and texts of yoga allows yoga therapists to translate between ancient wisdom and the modern context of their clients. We can consider the symbolism offered in the stories, listen deeply to the client's own narrative and needs, and discern how to best apply the philosophical foundation to an individualized practice for balance and well-being.

Personal Transformation

The *Bhagavad Gita* exemplifies one of these powerful stories through which we can explore certain themes, common to many yoga traditions and texts, in their applications to yoga therapy. The Bhagavad Gita illustrates a yogic path of transformation.

The Bhagavad Gita is part of a larger story called the *Mahabharata,* an epic that arose from the oral tradition. The Mahabharata is a prime example of a fluid narrative that evolved as stories, including the Bhagavad Gita itself, were added.[3] Both works offer a multitude of anecdotes on the situations that inevitably arise on the journey through life and through which practitioners may consider yoga's teachings.

The Mahabharata tells the story of a group of brothers, the Pandavas. Each brother represents essential parts of ourselves, including the ways in which we respond and orient to circumstances and events. We must recognize and understand each of these aspects of ourselves to effectively work with the vast array of body, mind, and environmental stimuli that arise throughout life. Central to these teachings is the idea that each experience may lead to or perpetuate an experience of suffering; alternatively, as we learn to find other ways to relate to these events we can find a greater sense of peace, contentment, and ultimately well-being in response to life.

Yudhisthira, the Pandava brother who is the son of Dharma, often plays the part of wisdom or the discerning mind. Bhima, the son of Vayu, the wind, represents will and strength. Arjuna is the Bhagavad Gita's main character and the archetypal warrior—the disciplined part of ourselves that demonstrates the utmost integrity in the face of any obstacle. As circumstances arise throughout the Mahabharata, we can see the response of each character and the strengths and weaknesses of their approaches to life. Interestingly, earlier sections of the text highlight the approach of Bhima, of strength and will; the central portion, including the Bhagavad Gita, concerns Arjuna, or discipline; and finally we turn to Yudhisthira, or dharma. Many will recognize the truth of experience in a path from the will with which we often approach life in our younger years to a more disciplined approach and ultimately one of greater wisdom and discernment as we mature.

The Bhagavad Gita's action takes place right before the central battle of the Mahabharata. This battle represents those moments in our lives when we face the turmoil of change and transformation and must work with whatever obstacles arise. When we arrive at these moments, our old ways and habits have taken us as far as they can; to change our relationship to suffering, we must confront whatever is limiting our progress. Arjuna represents our discipline to approach transformation with strength and wisdom.

The Bhagavad Gita begins with the scene of battle being described to a blind king, Dhritarastra. Leading up to this conflict, the king had many opportunities to see the truth, speak up, and take action that could have prevented the suffering that arose in the story of the Mahabharata. Instead, he was blinded to the truth and unable to discern the right actions to take, his vision clouded by emotions and beliefs he was unable to face. Dhritarastra plays the part of ourselves that has been blinded to understanding of what must be done to alleviate suffering or bring about peace. He comes to the battle from this clouded place, able to watch what happens only through another, who helps him "see" clearly. This partnership between the king and his advisor reminds us that when we bring ourselves to battle to confront a truth, we must often rely on others for support. In times of challenge, those we trust may support us by offering clear sight along our path.

This teaching is relevant today as we learn the importance, to health, of social relationships and connection. Historically, the biomedical explanatory model has underemphasized the social aspect of health, although its importance is gaining recognition. Chapters 6 and 7 of this book elaborate on the connection between this social dimension and health and well-being in terms of both physiological and psychological mechanisms and implications for yoga therapy. From the yogic perspective, the concept of connection is essential to the alleviation of suffering.

As the moment of battle arises, Arjuna comes to the middle of the field to look at both sides. He regards the "wrongdoers" who have acted in ways full of jealousy, arrogance, and greed—against everything that is "right." In them, Arjuna sees his teachers, uncles, cousins, and friends. He realizes he will have to fight those who have supported and taught him, those he has loved and been loved by. At the crossroads of transformation, we will encounter aspects of ourselves that have served us but that we now have to let go. Ways of thinking, beliefs we have held, and ways of understanding ourselves and the world that have kept us safe will shift in this process of change. In the same way that Arjuna realizes he will have to fight these people who have brought him so much, transformation brings the realization that our old ways of being may need to fall away to allow space for change. The beliefs that strengthened us at one time may be the very ones limiting us. Our work to alleviate suffering—or to change our relationship to its nature—may entail a release of the identity to which we cling.

When Arjuna realizes that this process of change includes parting ways with and "killing" friends, family, and teachers, he falters. He turns to Krishna, who represents the highest expression of teacher and spirit within, and laments:

> My limbs sink, my mouth is parched, my body trembles…I cannot stand still, my mind reels…I do not want to kill them even if I am killed…The

greed that distorts their reason blinds them to the sin they commit in ruining the family, blinds them to the crime of betraying friends.

(Bhagavad Gita, 1.29–1.38)[4]

Arjuna collapses in the middle of the battlefield, unable to discern next steps or even to distinguish right from wrong. Illustrating the difficulty in facing our safely established habits, this moment represents a decision point in the process of letting go patterns that perpetuate suffering and of choosing another way of being in relationship to life—so that we experience well-being and alleviate our suffering.

Each opportunity for change and growth brings corresponding obstacles in the form of "safe," perhaps long-held, patterns that challenge transformation. We must be ready to shift those beliefs if we are to move toward truth, meaning, and well-being. As these old patterns and beliefs fall away, we may become overwhelmed by the enormity of what may feel like insurmountable obstacles to change. These decision—and action—points are powerful opportunities to experience the truth of who we are without our fears.

The teachings of yoga are meant to assist us in this transformation. This wisdom tradition provides a map with which to traverse the path toward realization and a means by which we can overcome obstacles to change our experience of suffering.

The overwhelming uncertainty that can cloud our judgment sets the stage in the beginning verses of the Bhagavad Gita. The rest of the text is a discussion between Arjuna and Krishna about the former's inner conflict. Throughout the Mahabharata, Krishna is nearly everyone's trusted advisor, the archetypal teacher within. Arjuna asks this teacher, this embodied form of spirit, the questions that arise as he wrestles with what to do. Krishna offers guidance to help Arjuna align with his path and right action.

The Bhagavad Gita's battle is the moment when we have worked diligently and with integrity but meet an obstacle that requires us to relinquish aspects of ourselves—parts with which we may identify deeply yet hold us back.

Practice 1.1 Meditation: Standing at a Crossroads

Take a few breaths and center your attention into your body. Recall a time when you experienced an obstacle and were unclear as to the truth or the direction to take. Notice how it felt to be at this crossroads.

> Allow the full experience of that moment to arise. How does it feel in your body to be at this decision point? Where in your body do you notice this obstacle, this questioning of which direction to go? What is the quality of sensation? Heavy/light, bright/dark, pin-pointed/diffuse? How do you notice in your body the experience of not being able to see clearly which direction to take? What thoughts, beliefs, and emotions emerge?
>
> What were your blindnesses at this crossroads? Were there practices that supported you in this or similar past situations when you experienced obstacles? How did you come to a decision and take action? How did that feel in your body? What thoughts, emotions, and beliefs supported that decision?

The Nature of Awareness

In working with clients, we will meet with people who are suffering. Their lives have been altered because of emotional and physical pain, illness, or disability. These changes bring people to a crossroads, where the ways in which they used to meet life may no longer be available or serve them. Identities may shift as the way the body functions, mental states or beliefs, and even social networks or available activities change.

If we consider the potentially transformative nature of pain, illness, or disability, yoga can help facilitate a process whereby the very relationship to life changes to lessen the experience of suffering and instead heighten well-being. To mitigate suffering, we can bring to the fore the qualities of equanimity, contentment, tranquility, and a steadfast expression of happiness stemming from the innate unity that lies within. Yoga's wisdom teachings have much to offer as we help clients meet, and shift the way they encounter, obstacles. The yoga therapeutic practice becomes a mechanism through which to explore habitual ways of responding to life and to find new relationships with the body, mind, and environment.

Yoga teaches a path that is meant to help the individual connect with unchanging awareness beneath the constructs of our bodily experience, thoughts, emotions, beliefs, personality, and even social or environmental contexts. Chapters 3 and 4 more completely define the constituents of material nature, such as the components of the mind, as distinct from awareness. Here, we explore unchanging awareness with its emergent experiences of equanimity, steadfast joy, and contentment. Yoga facilitates connection to this unchanging internal recognition to mitigate suffering.

The direct experience of awareness is essential to achieve liberation from suffering. Yoga therapy, rooted in this philosophical foundation, intends to help individuals reconnect to underlying awareness. The yoga therapist's focus is not the medical diagnosis or condition of the client. Rather, her process facilitates an unpeeling of the layers that obscure the recognition of equanimity, steadfast joy, or contentment; in the therapeutic relationship, the yoga therapist and client walk a journey together, creating space for the connection to awareness to unfold.

An Individualized Shared Language

Speaking meaningfully about the idea of awareness can be difficult in healthcare contexts. We may even be uncomfortable discussing such concepts, which can seem nebulous at first, with clients. However, we can work with ideas of unity or reconnection alongside the experience of steadfast equanimity and contentment while honoring each person's unique path and beliefs.

One client wanted to learn yoga but was guarded because she felt she would be working with spirituality outside the existing framework of her strong religious beliefs. She was torn, as she wanted to explore her connection to suffering and well-being while honoring her belief system. We discussed ideas of spirituality, including the attributes of equanimity, contentment, steadfast joy, and compassion, and how she connects to and understands these concepts. She shared with me her relationship with Christianity. We were able to create a common language to work with her pain and suffering and to explore her relationship to life through the beliefs that held personal meaning for her.

I have worked with others for whom the language of neurophysiology provided the translation needed to speak to this connection. In my experience, once a shared language is found, people become receptive to how yoga can help them in alignment with their own beliefs and needs. Given an appropriate shared language, the concept of connecting to another layer of who we are beneath our pain is accessible to most and can be done with respect of each individual's experience of unity.

Being in conscious relationship to awareness underlying our day-to-day experience is the core of an explanatory framework of yoga therapy; rather than shying away from a discussion of this concept, we need to find accessible ways to describe and teach it. Key to this framework is the concept that who we truly are differs from the subjective reality we are experiencing. How do we find unifying language to speak to this concept and allow everyone space for their individual beliefs? How do we reliably use this shared language to express the nature of awareness? How do we make these ideas accessible? Throughout this book, my intention is to share these different ways of articulating the wisdom of yoga for use in both research and clinical contexts.

When Arjuna is overwhelmed by confusion and doubt about the correct path, Krishna offers this teaching on the nature of unchanging awareness:

> Indestructible is the presence that pervades all this; no one can destroy this unchanging reality. Our bodies are known to end, but the embodied self is enduring, indestructible, and immeasurable...
>
> (Bhagavad Gita, 2.17–2.18)

> It is not born, it does not die; having been, it will never not be; unborn, enduring, constant, and primordial, it is not killed when the body is killed.
>
> (Bhagavad Gita, 2.20)

> It is called unmanifest, inconceivable, and immutable; since you know that to be so, you should not grieve!
>
> (Bhagavad Gita, 2.25)[5]

This teaching is also found in the Upanishads:

> Beyond cause and effect, this Self is eternal and immutable...Hidden in the heart of every creature exists the Self, subtler than the subtlest, greater than the greatest....
>
> (Katha, 1.2.18–1.2.20)

> As the same air assumes different shapes when it enters objects differing in shape, so does the one Self take the shape of every creature in whom he is present.
>
> (Katha, 2.2.20)

> The Self is the source of abiding joy...When one realizes the Self, in whom all life is one, changeless, nameless, formless, then one fears no more. Until we realize the unity of life, we live in fear.
>
> (Taittiriya, 2.7.1)

> As a lump of salt thrown in water dissolves and cannot be taken out again, though wherever we taste the water it is salty, even so, beloved, the separate self dissolves in the sea of pure consciousness, infinite and immortal. Separateness arises from identifying the Self with the body, which is made up of the elements; when this physical identification dissolves, there can be no more separate self.
>
> (Brihadaranyaka, 2.4.12)[6]

These teachings describe awareness as an eternal presence within that cannot be harmed or changed and that differs from our changing experience of the body, mind, or environment. The experience of these phenomena can unfold in awareness without identification or fusion with them. This understanding is paramount in exploring the meaning of suffering and working toward its alleviation. Connecting to awareness is an essential foundation for the yoga therapy framework.

The concept of a steadfast, unwavering equanimity and contentment that emerges from connecting to awareness in any moment can be esoteric or incredibly practical and tangible. We can ask clients about their understanding of concepts such as soul or spirit. We can also look to the texts above, which describe awareness as imbued with connection, joy, and unity. Delving into a process of inquiry with clients about an experience of connection to another person, some other being, or with the world, may help them to embody this concept. Asking about an experience of joy or unity may initiate a process of remembering an aspect of themselves that lies beneath their pain or suffering.

Glimpses of this realization remind us that separateness is an illusion; our journey to recognize innate unity is the truth. Embodying unitive awareness gives rise to steadfast and unwavering joy amidst the fleeting phenomena of body, mind, and environment. Helping people experience this is a way to speak to the spirituality and connection inherent within us. Clients working with me have described this experience in many ways, including visually as colors like blue or bright violet; as feelings of expansion or lightness; as a being that supports them; as their favorite animal; and in words like peace, love, or compassion.

Although awareness can represent a challenging exploration, it is essential to define as the foundational concept in our yoga therapy process; we are working to facilitate this very experience of connection, equanimity, contentment, and steadfast joy within. Moreover, we will begin to explore how such experiences bring about potentially important physical and mental health benefits. Understanding some of the neurophysiological mechanisms underlying these effects can help us to open a dialogue with clients and help them find their own language for expressing these experiences. Note that a discussion of physiology is not meant to reduce spirituality to physiological processes, but rather to offer another door through which clients may become comfortable with concepts of connection, joy, and so on.

Eudaimonic Well-Being and Meaning

The concept of aligning with unchanging joy can be found in Aristotle's teachings. For him, *eudaimonia* results from a life well-lived and well-intentioned. Eudaimonia is reaching one's potential as an "excellent" and pinnacle example of a human life.[7]

This philosophical perspective includes a definition of two types of happiness: eudaimonic and hedonic. *Eudaimonic happiness* is independent of momentary events, steadfast, and enduring—similar to contentment, or the niyama of *santosha* in yoga. On the other hand, Aristotle describes *hedonic happiness* as pleasurable and transitory experiences that arise and fall away quickly. The qualities that emerge from the yogic description of awareness—equanimity, steadfast joy, contentment—align well with the features of eudaimonic happiness.

Yoga's potential to facilitate qualities of eudaimonic well-being is significant considering the research on the health benefits described below. Research considers eudaimonia through concepts such as self-actualization, flourishing, optimal functioning, and connection to purpose and meaning. Hedonic happiness is more analogous to emotional health, often described as happiness or cheerfulness.

Eudaimonic well-being is associated with positive health outcomes—including improved immune function, decreased inflammation, decreased allostatic load, and decreased all-cause mortality (see Chapter 6 for more details)—independent of variables such as age, disease, and physical inactivity.[8] Eudaimonic well-being measures, such as reported connection to meaning and purpose, are correlated with downregulation of gene expression profiles that affect inflammation and immune function and are important in many conditions, including cardiovascular and neurodegenerative diseases and cancers; hedonic well-being has been shown to upregulate these same gene profiles.[9] In other words, our human genome is sensitive to whether our experience of well-being is steadfast or transitory, eudaimonic or hedonic, and engages distinct patterns accordingly. These patterns of genetic expression can either move us toward or away from greater health in response to stress or adversity. All of this highlights the importance of eudaimonic well-being for physical and mental health, irrespective of other factors. Yoga therapy's foundation in facilitating realization of awareness, through which attributes that parallel eudaimonic well-being (steadfast joy, contentment) emerge, makes it an exemplary methodology for whole-person health and well-being.

Offering another perspective that emphasizes the importance of connection to meaning or purpose, psychiatrist and psychotherapist Viktor Frankl writes, "In some ways, suffering ceases to be suffering the moment it finds meaning." According to Frankl, author of *Man's Search for Meaning*, the experience of suffering, regardless of circumstance, can be lessened by cultivating meaning and undertaking right action to fulfill that meaning. Frankl's teachings emphasize that finding meaning is not an abstract, esoteric concept, but rather a tangible way to decrease suffering.

Eudaimonic and Hedonic Happiness in Yoga Therapy

Yoga therapy can provide powerful practices to facilitate these experiences of meaning, purpose, and steadfast joy. As we elucidate the explanatory framework of yoga therapy in health and disease, we will explore this perspective of helping clients change their understanding of and relationship to suffering by finding meaning, purpose, and right action. The yoga therapist is uniquely situated to facilitate a process in which—regardless of condition, illness, or pain—the primary focus is the cultivation of eudaimonic well-being rather than simply hedonia, alleviation of pain, or improvement of function.

The Upanishads offer teachings that further differentiate eudaimonic from hedonic experience:

> In the secret cave of the heart, two are seated by life's fountain. The separate ego drinks of the sweet and bitter stuff, liking the sweet, disliking the bitter, while the supreme Self drinks sweet and bitter neither liking this nor disliking that. The ego gropes in darkness, while the Self lives in light. So declare the illumined sages….May we light the fire of Nachiketa that burns out the ego and enables us to pass from fearful fragmentation to fearless fullness in the changeless whole.
> (Katha, 1.3.1–1.3.2)

> Like two golden birds perched on the selfsame tree, intimate friends, the ego and the Self dwell in the same body. The former eats the sweet

and sour fruits of the tree of life while the latter looks on in detachment. As long as we think we are the ego, we feel attached and fall into sorrow. But realize that you are the Self, the Lord of life, and you will be freed from sorrow. When you realize that you are the Self, supreme source of light, supreme source of love, you transcend the duality of life and enter into the unitive state.

(Mundaka, 3.1.1–3.1.2)[10]

These two excerpts point to the profound difference between transitory and steadfast joy—hedonic compared to eudaimonic—in the yogic tradition. Yoga teaches us that once situated in the recognition of awareness, we can experience the pleasant and unpleasant, the sweet and bitter, yet continue to take in the fullness of life and connection to the whole. We can find a different way of being in relationship to the ever-changing phenomena of the body, mind, and environment, a shift from the experience of suffering to the experience of unity and fullness. Being established in eudaimonic happiness offers a way to move from fear, disconnection, and sorrow toward wholeness, irrespective of the transitory occurrences we experience. The practices and teachings of yoga are meant to help us realize awareness so our very reactions to external events change. In other words, we can be present to the myriad experiences of life and continue to rest in a foundation of steadfast joy, or eudaimonic well-being, that lies within.

Hedonic happiness—the domain of the ego rather than the Self—is instead a grasping in darkness for one thing and then another, a constant search for the pleasant and fear of change and the unpleasant. (The ego and related concepts, both yogic and contemporary, are discussed in Chapter 4.) The hedonic experience is one of continually running away from something we think brings us sorrow and toward something that feels good. This incessant pull creates fragmentation and can never lead to satiety. Yoga teaches us about our capacity to abandon hedonic drives and find another way to meet life and its multitude of experiences. The Bhagavad Gita says,

> The joy of lucidity at first seems like poison but is in the end like ambrosia, from the calm of self-understanding. The joy that is passionate at first seems like ambrosia when senses encounter sense objects, but in the end it is like poison.
>
> (18.37–18.38)[11]

The clarity that comes with connection to and realization of awareness may initially seem difficult or like a withdrawal from certain pleasures but in the end represents a deep, abiding, and steadfast joy. The momentary pleasure of transitory happiness, on the other hand, ultimately leads to dissatisfaction and may even be detrimental.

This shift in relationship to life's occurrences allows clients to understand their own suffering; to see the many ways in which they meet body, mind, and environmental phenomena so as to perpetuate this suffering; to change suffering as they come into alignment with meaning and purpose; and ultimately to experience the qualities of equanimity, eudaimonic well-being, and contentment that emerge from the realization of awareness. This understanding that there exists another way to navigate life is at the core of the yoga therapeutic process.

Conclusion

The realization of awareness with its emergent properties of equanimity, eudaimonic well-being, and contentment is the crucial intention toward which yoga's practices orient. Rather than treating a constellation of symptoms associated with low back pain, anxiety, or diabetes, we have a methodology to reconnect people to unitive awareness from which they can experience eudaimonic well-being, with its physical and mental benefits. This approach helps the client with low back pain realize that her musculoskeletal imbalances are potentially rooted in how she meets external stimuli in ways that perpetuate tension and pain, while empowering her to change such patterns. Similarly, the person with anxiety or diabetes can experience deep peace and relaxation—with all of the physiological and mental benefits of such states—and understand how his habitual reactions maintain imbalance.

This book explores eudaimonic well-being as a useful way to bridge healthcare and research contexts to yoga therapy's intention to facilitate a connection to unchanging awareness. The attributes of eudaimonic well-being, equanimity, and contentment emerging from the realization of awareness, and their benefits to health and well-being, provide a context for the practices of yoga therapy and define the perspective of the yoga therapist. Throughout the book we will continue to consider the neurophysiological underpinnings of eudaimonic well-being, its effects on mental and psychological health, and practical yoga therapy applications to help facilitate its experience.

Practice 1.2 Meditation: Remembering Connection and the Unity With Awareness

Settle into your body, spending a few moments noticing the rise and fall of the breath. Think of a time when you felt safe and content, connected, joyous, or loved, in alignment and union with all that surrounded you. Perhaps during a period of quiet reflection in nature, or in a gathering of family or friends where you were completely at ease. If no occasion arises, you might simply imagine a feeling of peace or connection. Allow the physical sensations of calm, however you experience them, to spread.

Allow a word or phrase that will symbolize that feeling to come into your attention. Offer that word or phrase to your whole body. First to your eyes, your head: "May you be filled with...ease, peace, love..." Offer this to your throat, neck, right arm, right hand, left arm, left hand. Offer this to your heart: With each inhalation fill the heart space with this intention, and with each exhalation feel how the heart space connects to and spreads this intention throughout your body. Offer this intention to your back, your abdomen, right leg, right foot, left leg, left foot. Offer this intention to each thought, emotion, and feeling that arises. Rest in this feeling and offering...

As you end your meditation, notice again the sensations present in the body. What is the physical feeling of connecting with ease, peace, love? Where and how do you notice it in your body? What types of thoughts or emotions are present?

What would it be like to navigate your life maintaining this connection to unity, joy, peace, connection?

Notes

1. Mallinson, J., & Singleton, M. (2017). *Roots of yoga*. London: Penguin.
2. Miller, R. (2015). From Level I training, Integrative Restoration Institute. San Rafael, CA: iRest Institute.
3. Doniger, W. (2010). *The Hindus: An alternative history*. New York: Penguin Books.
4. Miller, B. S. (Trans.) (1986). The Bhagavad-Gita: Krishna's counsel in time of war. New York: Bantam Classics.
5. Miller, B. S., *The Bhagavad-Gita*.
6. From *The Upanishads* (Vol. 2), translated by Eknath Easwaran, founder of the Blue Mountain Center of Meditation, copyright 1987, 2007; reprinted by permission of Nilgiri Press, P. O. Box 256, Tomales, CA 94971, www.bmcm.org.

7. Aristotle. (2004). *The Nicomachean ethics*. (J. A. K. Thomson, Trans., & H. Tredennick, Further Rev. Ed. Trans.). London: Penguin Books.
8. Cole, S. W., Levine, M. E., Arevalo, J. M. G., Ma, J., Weir, D. R., & Crimmins, E. M. (2015). Loneliness, eudaimonia, and the human conserved transcriptional response to adversity. *Psychoneuroendocrinology, 62*, 11–17; Keyes, C. L., & Simoes, E. J. (2012). To flourish or not: Positive mental health and all-cause mortality. *American Journal of Public Health, 102*(11), 2164–2172.
9. Cole et al., Loneliness, eudaimonia and the human conserved transcriptional response to adversity; Fredrickson, B. L., Grewen, K. M., Coffey, K. A., Algoe, S. B., Firestine, A. M., Arevalo, J. M. G., ... Cole, S. W. (2013). A functional genomic perspective on human well-being. *Proceedings of the National Academy of Sciences, 110*(33), 13684–13689.
10. Easwaran, *The Upanishads*.
11. Miller, B. S., *The Bhagavad-Gita*.

Dharma, Ethics, and Right Action

2

Nearing the end of a period of exile in the forest, the five Pandava brothers find themselves in dire need of water. The eldest, Yudhisthira, sends his brother, Nakula, in search of water. After a time, Nakula comes upon a shimmering lake filled with vibrant lilies and lotuses. Eager to quench his thirst and gather water for his brothers, he rushes toward the lake. A booming voice surrounds him: "Do not take this water. It is my property, and taking it without permission is an act of violence. Answer my questions first, and then you may have as much water as you would like."

Nakula, desperate for a drink, does not heed this warning. Upon tasting the water, he collapses on the lake shore. Eventually, when Nakula does not return, Yudhisthira sends another brother in search of Nakula and of water. One by one, each brother leaves to find water and, disregarding the voice's warning, succumbs to his thirst and collapses beside the lake.

When none of his brothers return, Yudhisthira, fraught with worry, goes in search of them. Upon seeing the glistening lake, he is overjoyed and rushes to the water. He then notices his lifeless brothers. Incredulous and distressed, he wonders who or what could have caused this calamity to befall his great and powerful family.

The booming voice addresses Yudhisthira: "Do not take this water without my permission. It is my property, and taking it without answering my questions is an act of violence. Your brothers did not listen to me and tried to take what is mine. If you answer my questions, you can have as much water as you like."

Yudhisthira, the son and representation of Dharma through the epic, replies, "I do not covet what is yours, nor do I wish to take what is not mine. We all must answer for our actions. I will answer your questions."

Yudhisthira satisfactorily answers each question—a dialogue that itself constitutes a wide-ranging discourse on wisdom, truth, and spirituality—and is given a reward of choosing one brother to revive. Surprisingly, Yudhisthira chooses Nakula rather than Bhima with his incomparable strength or Arjuna with his legendary warriorship.

Yudhisthira offers his reasoning: "Nonharming and noncruelty are the highest of virtues, which I will always uphold. When we sacrifice this virtue we sacrifice ourselves, and so I will not violate this. I will not harm, nor will I be cruel—Nakula shall live." The brothers, all raised together, were born of two mothers, and Yudhisthira explains that it would be cruel to allow only sons of Kunti—himself, Bhima, and Arjuna—to live. The choice of Nakula, a son of Madri, gives both mothers surviving offspring and thus upholds the virtue of nonharming.

Because Yudhisthira values nonharming above profit or pleasure, he is given another reward—all of his brothers will be restored to life. Dharma reveals himself to be the one who has been questioning Yudhisthira, saying he wanted to come and see his son, and to test him. Dharma is pleased at his son's commitment, understanding, and application of nonharming and grants him three more favors. For the final favor, Yudhisthira asks for the virtues of good character such as an ability to overcome anger and a mind devoted to charity, truth, and austerity.

Dharma grants him these virtues, then explains that merits like truth, self-control, purity, uprightness, modesty, steadfastness, and charity constitute dharma itself. The doorways through which one can enter into dharma include the practice of virtues such as nonharming, noncruelty, freedom from malice, equanimity, tranquility, and purity.

Adapted from translations by J. A. B. van Buitenen,
K. Ganguli, and K. Dharma[1]

Dharma: A Framework for Action and Pinnacle Human Aim

The characters of the Mahabharata are presented with various situations that ask them to grapple with the enigma of dharma. In *The Hindus: An Alternative History*, Wendy Doniger writes that the epic helps to both "deconstruct" and "problematicize" dharma. Dharma is described as a subtle, malleable, inconsistent, and vague construct[2]; its nuances and fluidity can only be revealed through practical application in the trials of life.

Life provides the ultimate testing ground for moving from an abstract theory of dharma to a meaningful and useful foundation from which to make decisions. Throughout the epic, the Mahabharata's characters are challenged to simultaneously uphold virtue and follow dharma in the face of complex, potentially problematic situations. These situations afford readers the opportunity to contemplate dharma's meaning as a practical philosophy of living.

The Sanskrit root of the word *dharma*—dhr, to sustain—sheds some light on its complex meaning.[3] Essentially, any endeavor that sustains both the individual and the world around her is a practice of dharma.[4] Richard Miller describes the word dharma from its root, ṛta, to be in harmony with the totality of the universe.[5] When our way of living is congruent with our dharma, we can sense the same feeling of harmony within ourselves as we align with universal harmony. These more general definitions are key to applying dharma across circumstances and over time. They help us to understand dharma as a pinnacle aim or intention from which to base conscious decisions. Moreover, considering dharma in this way helps us to undertake actions that support ourselves within a context of harmony that extends to others and the surrounding environment.

A Guide to "Right Action"

Dharma provides a backdrop through which we can foster the discernment to determine the right action to take in response to life situations. Each time the characters of the Mahabharata are presented with a problem and have difficulty discerning right action for the given context, they are advised to take the action that will benefit, support, or sustain both themselves and the world.[6] These stories provide concrete examples to help us move from abstract ideas of what might be "right" or "good" in a given situation to practical application of dharma. Each instance clarifies the alignment with dharma that guides right action.

Practicing virtues and ethical qualities such as nonharming, equanimity, and tranquility is taught as a way to actualize the harmony of dharma, as demonstrated in the story at the beginning of this chapter. These virtues form intentional practices that can direct us toward action that supports the realization of dharma.[7] In yogic teachings, the yamas and niyamas essentially comprise the practice of these virtues in reference to interaction with oneself and the world. For example, working with the yama of *ahimsa* may mean asking a client to explore what it means to be nonharming to the body, mind, and other beings. In this way we can create an embodied, applied meaning of these virtues, or ethical practices.

> **Practice 2.1 Virtues and Dharma**
>
> Sit in a comfortable and relaxing space with a journal or piece of paper. Take a few breaths and elongate the exhale. Notice the body, scanning from the top of the head to the feet. Note any areas of tension and slowly cultivate an intention to relax these areas; allow each exhalation to help release tension.
>
> Dharma is that which sustains you and the world around you. It is experienced as both inner and outer harmony and is comprised of such characteristics as truth or steadfastness. What do these concepts mean to you?
>
> Choose one or two of these ideas:
>
> - truth;
> - steadfastness;
> - that which supports and sustains you and the surrounding world; or
> - inner and outer harmony.
>
> What does it feel like to connect to these concepts in this moment? Where do you notice them in your body? Is there a color or image that presents itself as the recognition of these characteristics? Breathe into that space of truth, steadfastness, sustenance, or harmony and allow it to become tangible—something that you can lean into and trust.
>
> Write down any notes about that space—words, images, affirmations.
>
> The practice of the virtues, including nonharming, equanimity, and contentment, helps to strengthen or reinforce dharma. Choose one of these virtues to explore. What is its feeling, shape, image? Where is it in your body? Let the quality you have chosen become tangible. What does it feel like? What happens to your muscles, posture, thoughts, emotions, and beliefs?
>
> Notice your relationship with yourself as you practice the virtues and align with dharma—that which supports and sustains you, inner and outer harmony. What would it mean to walk around for a day embodying the characteristics of dharma and the qualities of nonharming, equanimity,

and contentment? What thoughts and beliefs would you hold? How would you interact with others? How would you speak? What would you do?

Over the next week, explore what it means to stay connected to this idea of dharma as that which sustains you, inner and outer harmony, and truth. Notice how the practice of the chosen virtue may assist in this alignment with dharma. Notice how this awareness affects you in terms of muscle tone and tension, postures, thoughts, emotions, energy levels, beliefs, and relationships with others.

Reconciling the Personal and the General in Dharma

Many yogic texts provide a roadmap of the steps that constitute a virtuous, fulfilling life leading to the actualization of dharma. A difficulty comes when the action being asked of an individual seems to be in opposition to upholding the virtues. The Mahabharata explores this question of reconciliation between one's actions and the virtues' highest aim: We are asked to grapple with what to do when right action opposes the ethical life, when satisfying one (right action in support of dharma) seems to violate the other (virtues like nonharming).

Because he is the son of Dharma, Yudhisthira's story throughout the text symbolizes this struggle between dharma and virtue. The lake story reveals that nonharming is the virtue Yudhisthira holds as his highest aim and intention, yet he takes part in a war that kills teachers, family, and friends. How could dharma or the virtue of nonharming be seen to be upheld through the actions of war? How does Yudhisthira, who holds nonharming in such high regard, come to terms with his harmful actions in the battle? How does one work with the subtlety of dharma?

Yudhisthira is tested many times to prove his commitment to nonharming and his understanding of the nuances of its application in various circumstances. First, in the story above, he chooses Nakula to live over his other brothers, who have been portrayed as more important to Yudhisthira's ultimate success. Another key test comes when Yudhisthira is about to enter heaven and refuses if he is not allowed to bring a dog that has served as his loyal companion. The dog reveals himself to be Dharma, and by choosing his canine companion over entrance to heaven Yudhisthira again demonstrates the virtue of nonharming. In his final test, Yudhisthira sees his brothers and wife in a hell-like realm. He chooses to stay and comfort them rather than going to heaven. Dharma is again pleased at his commitment to and proficiency at both understanding and practicing nonharming.

Although he successfully demonstrates practical understanding of nonharming in these instances, Yudhisthira struggles with the decision to go to battle and whether it violates his commitment to this virtue. Yudhisthira seeks the advice of Bhishma, a great warrior and counselor, to resolve the conflict between actions deemed necessary for the sustenance of the world in his role as a king and his commitment to nonharming. Bhishma advises him on discerning between a general, abstract ideal of dharma and one's own individual dharma. Dharma and the virtues that lead to it always include that which sustains the individual and the world, but the action needed in a particular circumstance can appear to be in opposition to fulfilling dharmic demands. This ambiguity of dharma and the virtues necessitates clarification through life circumstances.

As a king, Yudhisthira's dharma is to take action to benefit his subjects and the world, even when that action conflicts with virtues such as nonharming. Bhishma encourages him to carry out his work as a king for the good of society. Through the roles we assume in the course of our lives, we have the opportunity to explore these virtues, or ethical qualities, and our own personal expression of dharma in relation to an abstract notion of dharma. Because Yudhisthira was presented with the responsibility of undertaking the role of king, he can be comforted in the manner in which he assumed that role and in how his actions benefited the whole of the kingdom.

Arjuna, too, is torn between his dharma—as a warrior—and the higher human aim of nonharming. At the moment of the start of the battle of Kurukshetra, Arjuna becomes unsure of being able to discern right action. Does satisfying dharma mean fighting his family and teachers and fulfilling his role as warrior? Or does it mean preserving his family and teachers and neglecting his role for the sake of nonharming? Which is the correct path of dharma that exemplifies the qualities of nonharming, equanimity, and contentment? Krishna counsels Arjuna that his dharma as a warrior is to fight; this action of battle is essential for the sustenance of the world and of Arjuna's family. As engagement in battle is the action being called for, undertaking it does not violate dharma or preclude a virtuous life. Krishna counsels Arjuna on the importance of one's personal dharma, saying, "Look to your own duty; do not tremble before it…"

Arjuna, a warrior, and Yudhisthira, a king, are both taught to apply virtues and dharma within the context of their life circumstances to help them fully grasp the meaning of these esoteric concepts. The fulfillment of dharma, and the virtues that lead to it, differ from one person and one situation to the next. Over and over, the reader is reminded that the practice of virtues is neither rigid nor black and white; living virtuously can be difficult and full of confusing contradictions.

Core virtues emphasized in the Mahabharata include truth, self-control, nonharming, equanimity, tranquility, patience, lack of anger, forgiveness, and kindness in thought, speech, and action.[8] These intentions form the foundation for the contemplation of right action in each circumstance so that dharma can be fulfilled even when a situation is complex.

Eudaimonic Well-Being: Another Practical Philosophy for Living

Chapter 1 introduced the concept of eudaimonia as a well-lived life, representing the pinnacle aim of being an "excellent" person. Eudaimonic well-being relates to a steadfast expression of joy, often differentiated from a transitory experience of (hedonic) happiness and conceptualized by meaning, purpose, flourishing, and self-actualization.

Central to yoga's teachings is the concept of awareness, from which features similar to eudaimonic well-being, such as steadfast joy, emerge. Moreover, because it includes ideas of meaning and purpose, flourishing, and self-actualization, eudaimonic well-being provides a significant parallel to concepts relevant to the discussion of dharma—actions promoting inner and outer harmony and those that sustain the individual in relationship to the world.

Another interesting parallel between yoga philosophy and the teachings of Aristotle is the emphasis on the virtues as a means to experience dharma and eudaimonia, respectively. As mentioned above, and according to Ananda Balayogi Bhavanani, the concept of dharma can be understood as responsibility for one's actions, which includes this alignment with the virtues.[9] Similarly, Aristotle teaches that eudaimonia results from acting in alignment with virtue—that "happiness is a certain activity of the soul in accordance with virtue."[10] Active, practical exploration guides us to apply the virtues to our own circumstances. Through this lens of ethical living, we can evaluate our actions, thoughts, and beliefs to discern a path of action leading to eudaimonia.

Just as yoga teaches that the practical application of the virtues in life is important to the realization of dharma, Aristotle taught the importance of the practical application of the virtues for the realization of eudaimonia. The exploration of these ethical principles allows each individual to apply the practices to their own circumstances to determine right action, leading to eudaimonia (Aristotle) or dharma (yoga).

Contemplating what brings about eudaimonic well-being—more specifically meaning, purpose, and steadfast joy—can help us develop insight for right action. This discernment in turn promotes healthy states of body and mind, as well as more positive relationships with others and the environment. We can gain clarity into those actions that cultivate eudaimonic well-being and those that lead us further away from it. The practices of the virtues are essential to this cultivation of eudaimonic well-being and dharma. As we access greater clarity through practice of the virtues we may shift away from habitual patterns that perpetuate suffering.

Engagement With the World

Many traditional sources of yoga emphasize the necessity of worldly experience for the realization of unchanging awareness. The Samkhya Karika (v. 57–61)[11] expresses that material nature (phenomena of body, mind, and environment) functions solely for the liberation of the spirit. As already discussed, the Mahabharata (and the Bhagavad Gita contained therein) also teaches the necessity of bringing yogic practices into the test of life so we can grasp their nuances. Only through the application of virtues and dharma in life's circumstances can we challenge our comprehension of these concepts.

Ultimately, each individual must reconcile the difficulties of living virtuously in the face of inevitable challenges; we dive into and actualize the meaning of the practices. The distinction between upholding these concepts in isolation and in relationship to the world and life events—philosophy in action versus intellectual endeavor—is vital in both yoga and Aristotle's teachings. Through the yamas and niyamas of yoga we can contemplate these virtues as a path toward dharma and eudaimonic well-being.

In the Mahabharata, the battlefield symbolizes the crossroads in life where one is asked to determine, amidst difficult circumstances, ethical and virtuous action that sustains and benefits oneself and others. These challenging moments call for discernment and proficiency in applying abstract concepts to real situations. Through the very obscuration of dharma or virtuous action we can grow in our understanding of these concepts. Anchoring to unchanging awareness and the emergent attributes of equanimity, eudaimonic well-being, and contentment facilitates the clarity from which to act in alignment with dharma.

Krishna tells Arjuna,

> When he...is content with the self within himself, then he is said to be a man whose insight is sure...
>
> (2.55)[12]

Being grounded in inner contentment strengthens the capacity for insight because this foundation connects us to awareness. From this connection, we can explore any situation and apply the virtues to realize eudaimonic well-being and dharma. Life experience helps us to develop the wisdom to distinguish actions that perpetuate suffering from those that align us with eudaimonic well-being and dharma. We can explore the actions that help cultivate deeper contentment, equanimity, steadfast joy, and inner and outer harmony—as distinct from those that lead us further from these qualities.

On the battlefield, when Arjuna begins to doubt whether he should act at all, Krishna is unequivocal. He teaches Arjuna not to relinquish his duty and to perform the action for which he is called. Rather than detaching or renouncing, the Bhagavad Gita asks us to engage in life for the fulfillment of our dharma:

> Perform necessary action; it is more powerful than inaction...
>
> (3.8)

> Renunciation and discipline in action both effect good beyond measure; but of the two, discipline in action surpasses renunciation of action.
>
> (5.2)[13]

Krishna teaches that necessary, right action is preferable to inaction or renunciation.

> What is action? What is inaction? Even the poets were confused—what I shall teach you of action will free you from misfortune. One should understand action, understand wrong action, and understand inaction too; the way of action is obscure. A man who sees inaction in action and action in inaction has understanding among men, disciplined in all action he performs.
>
> (Bhagavad Gita, 4.16–4.18)[14]

The reader is being asked to contemplate the differences among action, inaction, and wrong action and to discern when action is inaction and vice versa.

Dharma and Virtue in Action

There are instances when we need to take action to support or help others, or ourselves, and we do not—action through inaction. I have worked with clients who understood that the source of their stress, pain, or suffering was a changeable and habitual way of relating to themselves or the world. Examples include not being able to "find time" to do an exercise, breathing practice, or meditation; how a person holds tensions in their body in response to others; and beliefs like never being "enough" or being unable to do anything about a situation or experience. As long as they continued these habits of either behavior or belief, their patterns of physical tension and the way they interacted in the world would be repeated—action through inaction.

We can support such clients in becoming ready to change by building recognition of their habits through journaling, meditation, inquiry, and introspection. We can also focus on building confidence and self-efficacy for change. The virtues, or yamas and niyamas, of truth, acceptance, patience, contentment, kindness, and nonharming are essential to this work. *Tapas,* a fiery quality of discipline and self-control, also helps clients appreciate and recognize their own inner strength to change.

I have also worked with people who seem to be taking lots of action through trying many different healing modalities but resist changing the deeper beliefs or relationships with life that are at the core of their suffering—inaction in the midst of action. Here again the support of virtues such as truth, self-control, steadfastness, patience, kindness, and equanimity have been key in helping these clients explore their resistance and foster specific right action.

The Bhagavad Gita teaches practitioners to shift their focus from the result of the action to the manner in which action is taken and to the action itself.

> Be intent on action, not on the fruits of action; avoid attraction to the fruits and attachment to inaction!
>
> (2.47)[15]

> Fixed in Yoga, perform actions....It is said that evenness of mind is yoga....Yoga is skill in action.
>
> (2.48–2.50)[16]

> Always perform with detachment any action you must do; performing action with detachment, one achieves supreme good.
>
> (3.19)[17]

The path of yoga is not a renunciation of or distancing from life—philosophy and action are not separate endeavors. Rather, yoga teaches equanimity in action. A shift in the focus underlying action allows us to gain insight and to undertake right action in alignment with virtues that fulfill dharma and eudaimonia. Furthermore, connecting to contentment, steadfast joy, or eudaimonic well-being in the midst of action allows us to explore patterns of reaction to the body, mind, and world that may perpetuate suffering.

On Meaning and Suffering

This shift in how we undertake action can be explored through the concept of *meaning*, which eudaimonic well-being also encompasses. As mentioned in Chapter 1, Viktor Frankl teaches that if it is to alleviate suffering, meaning must be concrete, action-oriented, and serve an individual's unique present-moment circumstances:

> For the meaning of life differs from man to man, from day to day and from hour to hour. What matters, therefore, is not the meaning of life in general but rather the specific meaning of a person's life at a given moment....One should not search for an abstract meaning of life. Everyone has his own specific vocation or mission in life to carry out a concrete assignment which demands fulfillment.
>
> (pp. 108–109)[18]

Frankl's emphasis on recognizing one's own specific meaning for one's unique circumstance mirrors Krishna's instruction. In the Bhagavad Gita, Krishna teaches Arjuna that it is better to perform one's own dharma than to try to do another's—the latter can create harm.

> Your own duty [dharma] done imperfectly is better than another man's done well. It is better to die in one's own duty; another man's duty is perilous.
>
> (3.35)

> Each one achieves success by focusing on his own action…Better to do one's own duty imperfectly than to do another man's well; doing action intrinsic to his being, a man avoids guilt. Arjuna, a man should not relinquish action he is born to, even if it is flawed…
>
> (18.45–18.48)[19]

Aristotle, Frankl, and yoga all teach a path of action in life for the alleviation of suffering. Aristotle and yoga emphasize the inquiry into virtues, whereas Frankl teaches the specific assumption of meaning to determine action.

The term *eudaimonic well-being* encapsulates these varied teachings to foster a way of meeting life with equanimity, contentment, steadfast joy, and meaning or purpose. The path of action formed in such states supports and sustains us, alleviates suffering, and promotes eudaimonic well-being itself.

Frankl describes a specificity of meaning that arises from life circumstance. Arjuna and Yudhisthira are likewise taught the specificity of dharma for each person and that life brings the opportunities to explore one's own personal expression of virtues and of dharma. Neither philosophy necessitates the projection of an externally generated meaning or dharma onto our lives. On the contrary, our life's meaning is offered to us through various circumstances. This understanding shifts the focus to exploring the present moment to cultivate eudaimonic well-being and dharma.

Frankl says,

> [I]t did not really matter what we expected from life, but rather what life expected from us…stop asking about the meaning of life, and instead… think of ourselves as those who were questioned by life…Our answer must consist, not in talk and meditation, but in right action and in right conduct. Life ultimately means taking the responsibility to find the right answer to its problems and to fulfill the tasks which it constantly sets for each individual.
>
> (p. 77; emphasis in the original)[20]

Meaning is revealed in our very engagement with life. Every experience, even those that create suffering, is an opportunity to explore concepts such as action in alignment with dharma. This moment-to-moment recognition of meaning and dharma comes from being present and responsible to life in a manner that facilitates connection to awareness and its concomitant eudaimonic attributes. From such an orientation to life we can inquire into the actions that both foster well-being and benefit those around us.

Yoga therapy facilitates this process as we help clients transform their relationship to phenomena of the body, mind, and environment. Dharma then becomes a practical enterprise, as Krishna tells Arjuna:

> The doors of heaven open for warriors who rejoice to have a battle like this thrust on them by chance. If you fail to wage this war of sacred

duty, you will abandon your own duty and fame only to gain evil.... could any suffering be worse?

(Bhagavad Gita, 2.32–2.36)

[T]he world does not flee from him nor does he flee from the world; free of delight, rage, fear, and disgust, he is dear to me.

(Bhagavad Gita, 12.15)[21]

When life presents the opportunity to actualize your path and navigate toward your dharma, it is an occasion to celebrate. Through the battle he faces, Arjuna has the opportunity to align with dharma (that which supports himself and the world) and the realization of unchanging awareness from which eudaimonic well-being, equanimity, and contentment emerge. By meeting life's obstacles—not by fleeing or avoiding them—we can actualize our dharma. These are opportunities for deeper insight from which eudaimonic well-being and steadfast joy can be realized. If we consider that Arjuna is killing his old beliefs and patterns that perpetuate suffering, he is faced with a choice of change: continue his patterns and suffer, or let these patterns go to find another way of navigating life, a path on which he is connected to a deeper aspect of himself. Arjuna is being asked to take responsibility and engage in life in a way that leads to the fulfillment of dharma and connects him to unchanging awareness. These teachings demonstrate the importance of both honest, dedicated inquiry and practical action as part of such a path.

For Aristotle, the ethical concepts are guideposts for well-aligned action. For Frankl, meeting life events with responsibility and finding the concrete, unique meaning of each situation mitigates suffering. In the Bhagavad Gita, remembering our dharma and connecting to unchanging awareness helps us to understand what action to take.

Yoga teaches a methodology that combines ethical inquiry, physical practices, breath, and meditation to develop the discrimination to identify right actions—those that lead to connection to unchanging awareness and thus the emergence of eudaimonic well-being. The Bhagavad Gita teaches that suffering arises when we do not understand, accept, or take responsibility for action in alignment with our dharma. This philosophy of engagement with life calls for us to be fully present to experience as a means of alleviating suffering.

Therapeutic Application

Illness, pain, or disability can shift one's sense of identity. A disconnect can develop between who we are in the present moment and who we were or

Dharma, Ethics, and Right Action   43

want to be. Clients can experience shifts in social connection, belief in their ability to fulfill intentions and purposes they held for their lives, and discord between who they are and who they want to be.

As their identity changes, clients' sense of meaning may shift as they may not be able to interact with life as they once did. Whereas in health the body is often in the background and transparent to experience, in illness the body may move to the forefront and become the lens through which life is experienced. Our field of attention may narrow so that all of life is filtered through this pain experience—relationships, work, and play can all fade into the background.

This shift in identity may create an experience of suffering as we come to terms with who we are in the present. The ideas of eudaimonic well-being, dharma, and meaning can help clients foster a different relationship to pain, illness, or disability. The changing contexts of life afford us the opportunity to explore right action to sustain and support ourselves and the world around us. Yoga therapy becomes a methodology to understand life's meaning within this context.

The explanatory framework of yoga therapy (discussed further in Chapter 6) describes this connection to both unchanging awareness and to eudaimonic well-being as a foundational experience from which we can shift habitual patterns of relating to the body, mind, and world. Yoga therapy enacts a process to help clients reconnect with meaning and unchanging awareness with its attributes of eudaimonic well-being, equanimity, and contentment regardless of their circumstances. The path of yoga helps clients reconnect with who they are outside their pain or illness experience, and provides a methodology to inquire into the nature of suffering. The illness experience then becomes an opportunity for exploring meaning, equanimity, the nature of awareness, and eudaimonic well-being, a point that cannot be overemphasized in describing a yoga therapist's role and scope of practice.

Yoga therapy works differently than allopathic medicine's diagnosis-driven model. Rather than one set of practices for a musculoskeletal condition, another for a psychological condition, and still another for a physiological condition, yoga therapy steps back to consider more broadly the whole being, the very nature of suffering, and inquiry into its alleviation. The yoga therapist co-facilitates a process by which the client explores these same questions. The yamas and niyamas of yoga can be a starting point for intentionally reorienting to what arises in the body, mind, or relationship to external circumstances. Through ethical inquiry, the person learns new ways of meeting thoughts, emotions, feelings, and sensations. For example, as a client is asked to consider the meaning of *nonharming* or *contentment,* she learns the habits of posture, muscle tension, thoughts, or beliefs that create pain or foster discontent. By holding a posture or way of thinking with contentment, she begins to shift the way she relates to what arises in her body, mind, or world. She may learn how many of her reactions and relationships to these stimuli are harmful or indicative of discontent, and how to shift to their opposites.

We can ask a client in pain to work with a shift in their own identification with physical, mental, and environmental phenomena to foster the qualities of eudaimonic well-being. This practice of ethical inquiry represents active engagement on the part of the client to redefine their own relationship to illness and pain to one that supports both the individual and those around them—a relationship that enhances meaning, value, purpose, and agency even in the face of change, illness, and pain. Working with the yamas and niyamas facilitates a reevaluation of life's meaning. This setting of intention, and its embodiment through yoga practices like asana and pranayama, are crucial in the shift toward a life well-lived.

Just as pain can reorient identity and meaning to create suffering, it can be a powerful motivator of change to facilitate reconnection to eudaimonic well-being. Discrimination and ethical inquiry can prompt a reevaluation of our relationship to the body, mind, and environment, and illness, pain, or disability can create the life challenge needed to practically implement these tools and realize eudaimonic well-being.

Practice 2.2 A Dharma Meditation Walk

Set aside some time for an unhurried walk outside.

As you move, feel the activation of the muscles that propel the body, the body's changing position in space, the constant shifts in the surrounding world. Deeply notice the physical experience of walking, along with your mental and emotional responses.

Pause at your halfway point before turning for home and consider how you might experience your travels differently when connected to attributes like meaning, purpose, inner and outer harmony, and unchanging awareness. Allow these attributes to become stronger, noticing how and where you feel and experience them in your body. Notice whether there is a word or image that helps you to affirm and make this experience more tangible. Let this feeling fill every cell and space in your body. Connection to these attributes can become the foundation from which all action taken aligns with dharma.

> As you continue on your walk, notice whether you can stay connected to these feelings and attributes. Notice how you would move and take in the world while connected to the experience of meaning, purpose, inner and outer harmony, unchanging awareness. Continue on your way, exploring how your experience shifts with this awareness.
>
> Notice when movement might disconnect you from this meaning, purpose, inner and outer harmony, and unchanging awareness—and how you return to it.
>
> As you end the walk, notice what you learned about moving and interacting in the world from this connection.
>
> As you go about your day, notice how you can always connect back to unchanging awareness, meaning, purpose, and harmony. Notice how that connection can shift your physical posture, including held tensions or perceptions of your body, and your thoughts, emotions, and interactions with others. Notice how your dharma—actions that supports you and those around you, inner and outer harmony—as well as meaning and purpose can become tangible.

Clinical Examples

"Chris" Was Experiencing Low Back and Sacroiliac Pain, Worry, and Anxiety

I asked Chris to settle into a sense of meaning and purpose. What did that mean to him? What did it look like? Feel like? He provided an image of a redwood tree running through the center of his body. Leaning into this image offered a sense of strength and wisdom.

We worked with strengthening that image, feeling it, and bringing it into different postures. First, we chose poses that helped him feel the image more strongly—*virabhadrasana* (warrior) I and II. Then we worked with postures that challenged these sensations. Chris worked with staying connected to strength in postures where weakness arose, which for him included restorative backbends like *supta baddha konasana* (reclining cobbler's pose).

Through carefully guided inquiry, beliefs arose: of not being strong enough in life, not being able to voice what he wanted. Chris practiced using the redwood image in his daily life, evoking it each morning and evening. This practice included visualization with postures that enhanced the capacity to feel the intention of strength in his body (e.g., warrior postures) and postures that challenged this felt sense (e.g., restorative backbends). His home practice was a means to strengthen his intention so that he could bring it into his life in circumstances that challenged his feelings of strength and ability to voice what he needed.

"Jade" Had Chronic Back and Hip Pain

Jade spoke of fear around new situations. We worked with what contentment or allowing would feel like, and the image she arrived at was that of an ocean. We strengthened the sensations associated with that image with postures that helped her to access allowing and contentment—in this case forward folds, which we modified to protect her back and hip by limiting the depth of the posture with bolsters and blocks. We then worked with postures that challenged Jade's ability to allow contentment and stay connected to the ocean within; for her, such poses included backbends and strong postures that require arm strength (e.g., plank, side plank).

Conclusion

Yoga teaches a path to align with unchanging awareness, a path through which equanimity, contentment, and eudaimonic well-being can be realized. This connection can inform action that supports cohesion with oneself, others, and the world. Dharma is a complex concept that embodies this alignment, guided by the ethical practices of the yamas and niyamas.

An active engagement with life can follow from this connection to awareness and the exploration of ethical practices that support our unique dharma. Yoga, Aristotle, and Frankl all teach that life constantly presents us with the opportunities to actualize meaning and identify right action. Through receptivity to life itself, we can dive into our circumstances in a manner that connects us to awareness with its emergent attributes of equanimity and eudaimonic well-being, which in turn changes our relationship to experience and ultimately the very nature of suffering.

The practices of yoga teach ways to identify habits, thoughts, emotions, and beliefs that obscure the clarity we need to actualize meaning, dharma, and eudaimonic well-being. Yoga can help us disentangle from those patterns that perpetuate suffering. The discernment and wisdom we cultivate helps us to meet life in a way that connects to meaning and purpose in each action. By honoring the life that arises, rather than blocking or shutting off from it, we find the anchor of purpose.

Our suffering arises from wanting the life in front of us to be different from what it is. Instead, if we work with what is present, we find our meaning within that very experience of life. When clients meet chronic conditions and explore meaning within the illness experience, their suffering may change. When I work with clients with diagnoses such as multiple sclerosis (MS), fibromyalgia, or chronic pain, we explore such concepts and work to help them remember who they are beyond their pain or illness. From a personal exploration of the virtues, dharma, and meaning within the context of their current condition, they can learn to identify the "right" action to better their lives—and the lives of those around them. The outcome is diminished suffering and enhanced eudaimonic well-being.

A gift of the stories of the Mahabharata and the complexity of these teachings is that they transcend time and place to be applicable to contemporary readers. Dharma and the virtue ethics are affected by a range of factors including one's current roles, stage in life, and societal environment; dharma shifts with circumstance. The stories highlight the ambiguities of dharma and the virtuous life and remind us that these ideas are meaningless in a vacuum—they must be applied to life and acted upon.

Notes

1. Dharma, K. (1999). *Mahabharata: The greatest spiritual epic of all time*. Badger, CA: Torchlight Publishing; Buitenen, J. A. B., van Buitenen, J. A., & Fitzgerald, J. L. (Eds.). (1973). *The Mahabharata: 2—The book of the assembly hall; 3—The book of the forest*. Chicago, IL: University of Chicago Press; Ganguli, K. M. (2001). *The Mahabharata* (Vol. 3). New Delhi: Munshiram Manoharlal.
2. Doniger, W. (2010). *The Hindus: An alternative history*. New York: Penguin Press; Raveh, D. (2016). *Sutras, stories and yoga philosophy: Narrative and transfiguration*. London: Routledge.
3. Embree, A. T., Hay, S. N., & De Bary, W. T. (Eds.). (1988). *Sources of Indian tradition* (2nd ed.). New York: Columbia University Press.
4. Embree, Hay, & De Bary, *Sources of Indian tradition*; Fitzgerald, J. L. (2004). Dharma and its translation in the Mahabharata. *Journal of Indian Philosophy, 32*(5–6), 671–685.
5. Miller, R. Personal Correspondence, April 13, 2018.
6. Embree, Hay, & De Bary, Sources of Indian tradition; Fitzgerald, Dharma and its translation in the Mahabharata.
7. Fitzgerald, Dharma and its translation in the Mahabharata.
8. Doniger, *The Hindus*; Fitzgerald, Dharma and its translation in the Mahabharata; Ganguli, *The Mahabharata*; Mallinson, J., & Singleton, M. (2017). *Roots of yoga*. London: Penguin; Smith, J. D. (Ed.). (2009). *The Mahabharata*. London: Penguin Classics.
9. Balayogi Bhavanani, A. (2017, May 9). The yoga of responsibility [blog]. Retrieved from https://moayush.wordpress.com/2017/05/09/the-yoga-of-responsibility/

10. Ostwald, M. (1962). *Aristotle: Nicomachean ethics*. Indianapolis, IN: Library of Liberal Arts.
11. Burley, M. (2007). *Classical samkhya and yoga: An Indian metaphysics of experience*. Abingdon, UK: Routledge; Bawra, B. V. (2012). *Samkhya Karika*. Ravenna, OH: Brahmrishi Yoga Publications; Miller, R. (2012). *The Samkhya Karika*. San Rafael, CA: Integrative Restoration Institute.
12. Miller, B. S. (Trans.) (1986). *The Bhagavad-Gita: Krishna's counsel in time of war*. New York: Bantam Classics.
13. Miller, B. S., *The Bhagavad-Gita*.
14. Miller, B. S., *The Bhagavad-Gita*.
15. Miller, B. S., *The Bhagavad-Gita*.
16. Sargeant, W., & Chapple, C. (1984). *The Bhagavad Gita*. Albany, NY: State University of New York Press.
17. Miller, B. S., *The Bhagavad-Gita*.
18. Frankl, V. E. (2006). *Man's search for meaning*. Boston, MA: Beacon Press.
19. Miller, B. S., *The Bhagavad-Gita*.
20. Frankl, *Man's search for meaning*.
21. Miller, B. S., *The Bhagavad-Gita*.

Foundations for Discernment

Understanding Prakriti, Purusha, and the Gunas

We have introduced yoga as a path of realization through which we can connect to unchanging awareness beyond the fluctuations of the body, mind, and environment. From this realization attributes of equanimity, eudaimonic well-being, and contentment may emerge. This process is taught as a path to the alleviation of suffering. Moreover, it is engagement with life, not its renunciation, that enables this intentional reorientation to circumstance. As a result, we can learn to meet life in a way that supports ourselves and those around us—actualizing dharma.

How does yoga facilitate this process of inquiry and realization? How does yoga help us to cultivate the discernment to observe ever-fluctuating phenomena while gaining insight into the causes of suffering and fostering eudaimonic well-being?

Samkhya and Its Relationship to Yoga

The philosophy of samkhya contains foundational concepts that are incorporated into yogic texts such as The Yoga Sutras of Patanjali and the Mahabharata, including the Bhagavad Gita.[1] Samkhya teaches a process of inquiry through which we can discover the difference between awareness and the body, mind, and environment. This chapter focuses on the samkhya and dualist teachings and perspective. Chapter 5 builds on this material to describe the nondual and tantric perspectives.

The Mahabharata and Bhagavad Gita emphasize that yoga and samkhya are two paths leading to the same goal. Yoga and samkhya share many teachings, including an emphasis on ethical principles such as compassion and nonharming, as well as the development of discernment for the realization of awareness and alleviation of suffering.[2] The two paths' approaches, however, differ. Yoga is more practical and experiential, and samkhya provides a theoretical approach of systematic inquiry.[3]

The term *samkhya-yoga* has been used to signify that yoga and samkhya are complementary philosophies that can be used together as a system of theory and practice.[4] Practitioners are provided with a way to explore their own experiences as practice and theory cultivate insight into habits, thoughts, emotions, and behavior to prompt recognition around the relationships and patterns that create suffering and how to work toward its alleviation.[5]

This chapter and the next explore key concepts from samkhya as they pertain to this inquiry into the nature of suffering. Building on the concepts already explored, the ideas of samkhya will help to fill out the explanatory framework of yoga therapy and its applications for clients. The Samkhya Karika is the focus of this information, as it comprehensively lays out the philosophy of samkhya. Other texts, as well as what I have learned from teachers and clients, supplement this material.

Purusha and Prakriti

Purusha and *prakriti* are key concepts taught in samkhya philosophy, where systematic inquiry into the distinction between these principles is the way to alleviate suffering.

The Bhagavad Gita describes purusha in the following way:

> Renouncing all actions with the mind, the masterful embodied self dwells at ease in its nine-gated fortress—it neither acts nor causes action.
>
> (5.13)

> Lacking all the sense organs, it shines in their qualities; unattached, it supports everything; without qualities, it enjoys them.
>
> (13.14)[6]

Purusha is the witness, spectator, seer, and enjoyer of all objects of materiality, including the body, mind, and environment. It is the principle of subjectivity, perceiving, and experiencing.[7] Purusha experiences all of the changes inherent to the material and manifest world but is free from entanglement with them; it neither acts nor resists action but is the pure witness to action. In the verse cited above, purusha sits within the fortress of the body with its nine openings to the outer world, portals through which it can experience environmental phenomena. This book uses the word *purusha* to convey the complex principle of the observer and experiencer of all that arises, moves, and falls away within the field of prakriti.

Prakriti encapsulates all of material nature including the body, mind (cognitions, beliefs, and emotions), and environment.

The Bhagavad Gita says of prakriti,

> The field denotes this body, and wise men call one who knows it the field-knower.
>
> (13.1)[8]

Prakriti is the principle of materiality, the "infinitely diverse creations witnessed" by purusha.[9] The Samkhya Karika includes mental processes, sense perceptions, and the capacity for interaction with the world as components of prakriti. Prakriti is both the range of psychophysiological components that make up the individual and the elements that make up the environment. As the concept includes both psychological and physical properties, defining prakriti as material nature is somewhat limited. This book uses the word *prakriti* to include the individual's psychophysiological processes and states as well as the material constituents of the environment in which we live.

> [K]now that anything inanimate or alive with motion is born from the union of the field and its knower.
>
> (Bhagavad Gita, 13.26)[10]

According to dualist samkhya, prakriti encompasses the field in which all ever-changing experience arises, be it physical or psychological, internal or external. Purusha is the immutable knower or observer of all that arises in this field, which is itself devoid of constituents or attributes. The inquiry of samkhya helps us understand that everything arises from this conjunction of purusha with prakriti. All things that change and shift are part of prakriti, not purusha; from this discrimination between the changing and the unchanging, we can begin to recognize unwavering awareness.

The Samkhya Karika says,

> The identification of Nature [prakriti] and Spirit [purusha] occurs solely within Nature...As long as these [predispositions of nature] are

engaged, misperception persists....The truth of the mistaken identification of Spirit and Nature is revealed by means of discriminative wisdom within the Intellect that seeks to understand the difference between Spirit and Nature.

(54)[11]

Through inquiry into the nature of the principles elucidated by samkhya, discriminative wisdom arises, enabling the distinction between purusha and prakriti. We begin to recognize that everything mutable—cognitions, emotions, beliefs, the body, and the environment—is prakriti, distinct from unchanging purusha.

When we confuse our identity with the changing attributes of prakriti, we suffer. Through the reorientation of our identity to purusha as an aspect of unchanging awareness, we are freed from enmeshment with prakriti. When we have the insight that prakriti and purusha are distinct, misperception ceases and liberation from suffering may occur.

Metaphors for Understanding Purusha and Prakriti

Metaphors adapted from the Samkhya Karika can help us apply its teachings to our own experience.

The Blind and Lame

> The proximity (or association) of the two, which is like that of a blind man and a lame man, is for the purpose of seeing the pradhana [original, undifferentiated material energy] and for the purpose of the isolation of the purusha.
>
> (Samkhya Karika, 21)[12]

> The union of Spirit with Nature is for contemplation of Nature; the union of nature with spirit is for liberation. The union of both Spirit and Nature is like that of a lame man with a blind man. The creation is brought about by that union.
>
> (Samkhya Karika, 21)[13]

Both principles—purusha and prakriti—are important. This metaphor emphasizes that their conjunction enables the end goal of liberation.

Here, a blind man and a lame man join together to complete a journey. Separately, they may not be able to successfully navigate this interaction with life, but together each benefits from the other's abilities. Likewise, purusha and prakriti come together for a mutually beneficial purpose. Purusha, like the lame man, is unable to move but can see; prakriti, like the blind man, can move but cannot see. The two properties of sight and movement must join together if they are to successfully reach the end of their journey. Mutually beneficial relationships emerge between perceiving (purusha), the individual and environment (prakriti), and engagement with life, providing experiences for this journey of liberation.

This teaching also clarifies that welcoming bodily and life experience enables us to gather insight. Just as the blind man and the lame man come together for the specific purpose of a journey, purusha and prakriti unite specifically for the contemplation of the body, mind, and environment. The opportunity to experience life gives rise to the potential for liberation from suffering. Indeed, we can only recognize purusha by experiencing prakriti's ever-changing attributes (body-mind-environment).

Viktor Frankl also emphasizes that receptivity to life provides the opportunity to create meaning in each moment and each circumstance:

> As each situation in life represents a challenge to man and presents a problem for him to solve, the question of the meaning of life may actually be reversed. Ultimately, man should not ask what the meaning of his life is, but rather he must recognize that it is he who is asked. In a word, each man is questioned by life; and he can only answer to life by answering for his own life; to life he can only respond by being responsible.
>
> (p. 109)[14]

Each life occurrence is an opportunity to explore meaning and to ultimately recognize the differentiation between prakriti and purusha. Life is always presenting us with the chance to connect to unchanging awareness within. By welcoming each occurrence, we can inquire into what is arising to realize this unchanging awareness in each moment. We do not have to try to create the right atmosphere for this to occur; every moment is an invitation for understanding. Rather than isolating ourselves or shutting off from life, bringing full, clear attention to what is being offered in every moment allows a choice of response. In our response to life, including what arises in the body and mind as well as outer circumstances, we find a crucial key for insight into the alleviation of our suffering.

The Dancer and the Dance

> Just as, having displayed herself before the gaze of the audience, the dancer desists from dancing, so prakriti desists, having manifested herself to purusha...In my view there is no one more tender than prakriti, who saying "I have been seen" never again comes into purusha's sight.
>
> (Samkhya Karika, 59–61)[15]

> Just as a dancer's performance reveals to the audience the story behind the dance, so liberation reveals the difference between Manifest Nature and Spirit. Upon liberation Nature, having served its ultimate purpose, ceases its binding performance of identification with Spirit. Nature, comprised as it is of the three constituents, appears benevolent and generous as it plays out its performance without benefit for itself. Spirit, in turn, being devoid of the constituents and incapable of being anything other than a witness of all that is performed by Nature, confers no benefit upon Nature. From the perspective of Samkhya there is nothing more creative, gentle, graceful, delicate, sensitive, and modest than Nature, which, knowing that "I have been seen," withdraws and never again engages in its prior role with Spirit as a binding force for misperception, ignorance, and suffering.
>
> (Samkhya Karika, 50–52)[16]

A dancer assumes a role to show the audience a story that is meant to help them understand a certain narrative or point of view; the performer's intent is to reveal something to the audience. Here, prakriti is likened to a dancer and purusha is the spectator.

Prakriti takes on various roles throughout an individual's life. Each role helps purusha to see itself as separate from these roles for the ultimate goal of realizing unchanging awareness and consequently liberating oneself from suffering. Just as the spectator of a dance can understand both the full story and the dancer's role within it, the roles of prakriti allow purusha the opportunity for this insight. Each story prakriti performs may end purusha's misidentification with prakriti.

Prakriti is said to engage with the story, or dance, solely for the purpose of demonstrating to purusha that the latter is the spectator rather than the story of the dance or the dancer. Once this is understood, the dance stops, having served its purpose; once purusha is no longer confused, prakriti is said to have served its purpose. When this insight happens, there are no more roles for prakriti to take on as purusha no longer misidentifies with the story and suffering ceases. Once this has happened, prakriti retreats and does not re-engage in the story. As prakriti assumes its roles without any intent of benefit to itself, it is described as gentle, benevolent, and modest, playing out a performance exclusively for the benefit of purusha.

The Potter's Wheel

> "I have seen her," says the spectating one; "I have been seen," says the other, desisting; although the two remain in conjunction, there is no initiation of [further] emergence. Due to the attainment of perfect knowledge, virtue (dharma) and the rest have no impelling cause; [nevertheless] the endowed body persists owing to the momentum of impressions, like a potter's wheel.
>
> (Samkhya Karika, 66–67)[17]

The potter's wheel that continues to turn after the pot has been removed is a powerful metaphor for what happens when purusha becomes free from misidentification with prakriti. This "liberation" does not mean that the engagement with life stops.

Once prakriti and purusha "see" and understand each other, there is no more confusion between them. Prakriti continues to move and engage with the world, but purusha can clearly distinguish between prakriti and itself. Changes in the physical body, psychological processes such as thoughts and emotions, and worldly interaction continue. However, the establishment of clarity between purusha and prakriti situates us firmly in the realization of unchanging awareness so that misperception no longer arises. The person can engage in life from this unshakable foundation of understanding unchanging awareness within.

Just as a potter's wheel continues to turn after the pot is removed, stimulus still arises in the body-mind, but purusha is no longer confused by it. We learn to notice habitual reactions and relationships and to interact with them differently. From the vantage point of a spectator, we can use the constantly changing experiences in the body, mind, and environment to connect to awareness. From this space, we can inquire into how to respond to life for the fulfillment of dharma and freedom from suffering.

Practice 3.1 Meditation on Purusha and Prakriti

First, journal about a difficult situation you have encountered. See whether you can relax around the details of the situation and write about how you felt in terms of:

- body sensation;
- thoughts, emotions, or beliefs that surface about yourself or your relationships with others; and
- your relationship or connection to the world.

Imagine this situation as a story, or dance, with yourself as the spectator. Notice the lines spoken as the players portray the situation. Notice the emotions conveyed through movement or words. Notice the story's similarity to others you have encountered.

Take a moment to thank this story for appearing, for showing itself to you.

Find a comfortable seat or lie down. Bring attention to the breath. Allow your attention to follow the rhythm and movement of breath.

Imagine your life experiences as opportunities to help you to realize unchanging awareness within, the unwavering seat of contentment, equanimity, and eudaimonic well-being. Each circumstance develops certain characteristics or ethical principles—trust, strength, compassion, patience—to help you realize that state of equanimity and contentment.

Connect to unchanging awareness that is within you at all times. How and where do you feel this in your body? Are there ways you could move to strengthen this feeling? Do any words or images strengthen this experience? Are there characteristics you could bring in to help you connect to unchanging awareness within…strength, trust, compassion, acceptance, patience? How can you strengthen these characteristics with movement, imagery, or words?

Come back to the story you are considering and again imagine yourself as a spectator. Can you watch the story and connect to awareness, or its qualities of contentment, equanimity, and steadfast joy? How would the characteristics of strength, trust, compassion, or acceptance be portrayed if they were meant to help facilitate this connection?

What needs to happen for you to cultivate these qualities that might allow you to remain equanimous as you watch this story unfold—are there images or words? How might you move to embody the strength or patience to connect to unchanging awareness within the context of this story? A warrior pose, standing balance, or a supported restorative backbend or forward fold? Explore those.

Return to your journal. What lessons can you learn from this situation to help you cultivate a connection to unchanging awareness within? What did you learn about the strength, patience, and compassion needed to connect to unchanging awareness?

As you write, notice if there is an image, word, or affirmation that helps to strengthen this lesson for you. What physical postures will enable you to practice embodying what you learned? How do you notice a felt sense of connection, of unchanging awareness? What are its characteristics? Is it in your belly, heart, whole body? Is it full, soft, strong?

Let this combination of intention with visualization or affirmation, posture(s), and felt sense be a meditation practice to strengthen the characteristics that help you experience the equanimity and steadfast joy of unchanging awareness within.

Prakriti and the Gunas

To assist practitioners in the process of inquiry and discernment, the Samkhya Karika elucidates the constituents of prakriti. Three substrates, the *gunas* of *rajas*, *tamas*, and *sattva*, combine to form all variations of the body, mind, and environment. In other words, the gunas' fluctuating proportions give all of prakriti its varied characteristics.

> The Three Constituents are different in their operation and makeup. Yet they function together for the ultimate purpose of the illumination and revelation of Spirit, just as the wick, oil, and flame of a lamp, though different in their makeup, function together for the purpose of illumination and revelation.
>
> (Samkhya Karika, 13)[18]

When different materials with their own specific properties are used together, as in a lamp, they can shed light on an object. Similarly, the gunas each have unique properties and work together to create body, mind, and environmental phenomena to illuminate the difference between purusha and prakriti. The three gunas combine with one another to support, modify, and generate all psychophysiological and environmental content. By understanding the gunas as part of prakriti, not purusha, we realize unchanging awareness within.

Sattva

> When the light of knowledge shines in all the body's senses, then one knows that lucidity prevails.
>
> (Bhagavad Gita, 14.11)[19]

Sattva guna is the substrate of calm, light, buoyancy, and illumination. From sattva, psychophysiological and behavioral experiences such as tranquility, harmony, equanimity, patience, joy, forgiveness, truth, contentment, humility, and compassion emerge. The capacity for clarity, discriminative wisdom, and virtuous or ethical behavior comes from being established in sattva. The predominance of this guna fosters the discernment needed to distinguish between purusha and prakriti.

This guna facilitates characteristics similar to those that arise from realization of unchanging awareness, so sattva can provide a glimpse into the unwavering equanimity of being firmly established in awareness. The cultivation of sattva plays an important role in the beginning of a practitioner's yoga practice, as this guna also helps to support the clarity needed to understand the other gunas, to discern between purusha and prakriti, and for the realization of awareness.

Rajas

> When passion [rajas] increases…, greed and activity, involvement in actions, disquiet, and longing arise.
>
> (Bhagavad Gita, 14.12)[20]

Raja guna is the substrate of energy, turbulence, and activity. The psychophysiological and behavioral characteristics that emerge from rajas include a spectrum ranging from excitement, motivation, and creativity to anxiety, arrogance, pride, anger, and agitation. This guna is vital in the capacity to move and create change; it underlies the practitioner's movement from habitual patterns to the development of new relationships with the body, mind, and environment. Although rajas' quality of agitation can cloud vision, it also provides the impulse and motivation needed for healthy engagement with life and the realization of awareness.

Tamas

> When dark inertia [tamas] increases, obscurity and inactivity, negligence and delusion, arise.
>
> (Bhagavad Gita, 14.13)[21]

Tama guna is the substrate of restraint, mass, and form. The psychophysiological and behavioral characteristics that arise from tamas include a spectrum that ranges from stability, groundedness, and boundaries to inertia, dullness, ignorance, and delusion. An unbalanced predominance of this guna in relation to the others promotes unvirtuous behavior, ignorance, and misperception. Tamas can obscure clarity, but it also creates the stability needed to support new behaviors and relationships with the body, mind, and environment for the alleviation of suffering and firm establishment in unchanging awareness.

The Gunas in Body, Mind, and Environment

The gunas reflect the dynamism inherent to all of life, including ever-changing physiological and psychological states and the environment. All thoughts, emotions, cognitions, and beliefs reflect the presence of the gunas in balanced or unbalanced distributions. Everything that comprises prakriti can be broken down into the proportions of its attributes of sattva, rajas, and tamas. From the predominance (imbalance) of rajas comes agitation, from tamas comes inertia, and from sattva comes clarity.

A healthy tree would reflect a balance of the three gunas with tamas in its solidity; rajas in its cycle of growth, maturation, and death; and sattva in its impassive equanimity. Leigh Blashki, yoga therapist and founder of the Australian Institute of Yoga Therapy, adds that sattva is the open receptivity of the tree's flower, which neither grasps nor rejects, but in its equipoise allows the essence of the tree to attract the creatures that pollinate it.

A healthy body would exhibit a mixture of the three gunas, reflecting the individual's nature and current circumstances with sattva in its vitality, rajas in its movement and activation of physiological processes (e.g., digestion, respiration), and tamas in its stability and form (e.g., skeletal structure). A preponderance of rajas may show up as high blood pressure or a stressed system with greater sympathetic nervous system activation (discussed in Chapter 7). Dominance of tamas could show up as fatigue or sluggishness.

A healthy, balanced emotional state would exhibit sattva in calmness or clarity, rajas in creativity or problem-solving ability, and tamas in focus or stillness. Excess rajas may show up as anxiety, anger, or fear, whereas excess tamas could show up as depression or confusion.

The Bhagavad Gita provides many examples of the psychophysiological and environmental characteristics that emerge from the gunas in their varying proportions.

Sattvic knowledge is described as when "one sees in all creatures a single, unchanging existence, undivided within its divisions" (Bhagavad Gita, 18.20).[22] On the other hand, rajasic knowledge sees only difference and separation between creatures, and tamasic knowledge "clings to a single thing as if it were the whole, limited, lacking a sense of reality" (Bhagavad Gita, 18.21–18.22).[23]

A sattvic person is one who "has no attachment...is resolute and energetic, unchanged in failure and success" (Bhagavad Gita, 18.26).[24] The rajasic person, however, is "anxious to gain the fruit of action, greedy, essentially violent, impure, subject to excitement and grief," and a tamasic person is "undisciplined, vulgar, stubborn...dishonest...and slow to act" (Bhagavad Gita, 18.27–18.28).[25]

As mentioned in Chapter 1, joy can take different forms. Sattvic joy is "like ambrosia, [arising] from the calm of self-understanding" (Bhagavad Gita, 18.37).[26] This joy, which arises from the realization of unchanging awareness—the understanding of one's essential nature—is similar to eudaimonic happiness. Rajasic and tamasic joy are similar to forms of hedonic happiness, described as tempting initially but then, respectively, as "like poison" and "self-deluding from beginning to end" (Bhagavad Gita, 18.38–18.39).[27]

Sattvic action "is necessary, free of attachment, performed without attraction or hatred by one who seeks no fruit" (Bhagavad Gita, 18.23).[28] Rajasic action is undertaken by one "who seeks to satisfy his desires," and tamasic action "is undertaken in delusion, without concern for consequences, for death or violence" (Bhagavad Gita, 18.24–18.25).[29]

Sattvic understanding is demonstrated by "one who knows activity and rest, acts of right and wrong, bravery and fear, bondage and freedom" (Bhagavad Gita, 18.30).[30] Rajasic understanding, however, "fails to discern... right acts from wrong," and tamasic understanding causes one to think "in perverse ways...covered in darkness" (Bhagavad Gita, 18.31–18.32).[31]

Sattva's Importance

Sattva guna underlies the understanding needed to assist practitioners in aligning with right action for the fulfillment of dharma. Action taken from the equanimity of sattva supports discernment and clarity so we can recognize what is needed to support the whole as well as the individual, to be in harmony with ourselves, others, and our environment. From a predominantly sattvic foundation, the virtues can be explored in a way that supports dharma.

Sattva shares many of the qualities—equanimity, contentment, eudaimonic joy—experienced in the realization of unchanging awareness. This glimpse of unwavering equanimity provided by sattva can be empowering and inspiring as it helps us to experience bodily sensation, thoughts, emotion, and the environment in a different way.

Through sattvic experiences, a person with chronic pain, anxiety, or depression discovers that it is possible to change the way they relate to physical or psychological stimuli. Eudaimonic well-being, contentment, and equanimity become accessible even amidst difficulty and pain. Yoga practices that promote sattva can be used to offer clients a tangible experience of equanimity so they relate to themselves and to the world differently. This can motivate continued practice and exploration of a different relationship with life.

As a clinician, I start from a viewpoint of nurturing the behaviors and the psychological and physiological states that build sattva. I help clients to more readily access the qualities that emerge from the experience of unchanging awareness—equanimity, connection, contentment, and eudaimonic well-being. Below, and in Chapter 9, we'll explore the use of postures, breath techniques, meditation, and ethical practices to encourage sattva and strengthen its experience to alleviate suffering.

Imbalanced Gunas, and Rajas and Tamas as Obstacles to Clarity

Bhishma's discourse to Yudhisthira emphasizes the cultivation of sattva, as both rajas and tamas can prevent clear sight. The equanimity of sattva prevents us from being overcome by the powerful forces of rajas and tamas.[32] Bhishma teaches that desire (rajas) is like a "tree growing in the heart," one whose "root can only be torn out by the sword of equanimity."[33]

62   Philosophical Foundations of Yoga

In a similar conversation, Arjuna asks Krishna what compels a person to do wrong. Krishna replies,

> It is desire and anger, arising from nature's quality of passion; know it here as the enemy, voracious and very evil! As fire is obscured by smoke and a mirror by dirt...knowledge [of the difference between purusha and prakriti] is obscured by this. Knowledge is obscured by the wise man's eternal enemy, which takes form as desire, an insatiable fire...
>
> (Bhagavad Gita, 3.37–3.39)[34]

Krishna calls rajas the main culprit obscuring discernment. Rajas underpins the emergence of characteristics such as anger, which prevent us from recognizing the difference between prakriti and purusha. Tamas likewise "obscures knowledge" (Bhagavad Gita, 14.9)[35] of this distinction.

Imbalanced rajas and tamas contribute to states of body and mind that limit the discernment needed for practitioners to realize and alleviate suffering. Most yogic texts highlight the dangers of rajas and tamas, but there is also a risk in trying to preserve sattva at the expense of acknowledging the inherent dynamism of life. Trying to stay in sattva can create avoidance, unhealthy attachment or detachment, or indifference. The concept of *spiritual bypassing* encapsulates this pitfall where, in the name of "spirituality," one does not engage with life, connect to others, or practice compassion and understanding. The Bhagavad Gita describes this situation by noting that sattva "binds one with attachment to joy and knowledge" (14.6) and "addicts one to joy" (14.9).[36]

The Gunas' Natural Dynamism

When the gunas are balanced, sattva promotes clarity for insight, rajas promotes motivation and creativity for right action, and tamas promotes stillness and stability for disciplined practice of yoga. Continual fluctuation of the gunas, however, is inherent to life. The body will always change in its state of health and even via natural aging processes. The mind will always shift from happiness to sadness, from to one emotion and thought to its opposite. The world continues to change as seasons shift and time moves on. Suffering arises from resisting change or not understanding that beneath this impermanence is a state of equanimity, connection, contentment, and tranquility. It is prakriti that changes, not purusha or unwavering awareness within.

Yoga teaches practitioners how to understand the rising and falling of sattva, rajas, and tamas and to connect to unchanging awareness within—to perceive the movement of the gunas and to connect to what is beyond, or beneath, that movement.

In the Bhagavad Gita, Krishna teaches Arjuna,

> When a man of vision sees nature's qualities as the agent of action and knows what lies beyond, he enters into my being. Transcending the three qualities that are the body's source [the gunas], the self achieves immortality, freed from the sorrows of birth, death, and old age.
>
> (14.19–14.20)[37]

When we see the gunas as the doers of all action, the movers within prakriti, we step into the realization of what lies beyond—awareness itself. By "transcending" the gunas we understand that we can experience their movement but are not them. This recognition of "something else" beyond the movement of the gunas is that of unchanging awareness. Realizing awareness, we can become free from the suffering that arises from misidentification with prakriti's continual shifting.

> As the mountainous depths of the ocean are unmoved when waters rush into it, so the man unmoved when desires enter him attains a peace that eludes the man of many desires.
>
> (Bhagavad Gita, 2.70)[38]

This metaphor captures the essence of transcending the gunas while remaining engaged with life: The ocean does not resist the movement of its waters, yet its depths remain unmoved by their surging. The unwavering equanimity that emerges from connecting to awareness can become an unshakable foundation from which to experience the waves of life's experiences.

Arjuna asks Krishna,

> [W]hat signs mark a man who passes beyond the three qualities? What does he do to cross beyond these qualities?
>
> (Bhagavad Gita, 14.21)[39]

Krishna answers,

> He does not dislike light or activity or delusion [the gunas]; when they cease to exist he does not desire them. He remains disinterested,

unmoved by qualities of nature; he never wavers, knowing that only qualities are in motion. Self-reliant, impartial to suffering and joy, to clay, stone, or gold, the resolute man is the same to foe and friend, to blame and praise. The same in honor and disgrace, to ally and enemy, a man who abandons involvements transcends the qualities of nature. One who serves me faithfully, with discipline of devotion, transcends the qualities of nature and shares in the infinite spirit. I am the infinite spirit's foundation, immortal and immutable, the basis of eternal sacred duty and of perfect joy.

(Bhagavad Gita, 14.22–14.27)[40]

When a person "passes beyond the gunas," she realizes unchanging awareness—beyond the fluctuations of body, mind, and environmental phenomena—and no longer misidentifies with the gunas or prakriti. By becoming firmly situated in this realization of awareness, she can fully experience the immense waves of the gunas but remain rooted in equanimity, impervious to being swept away by the phenomena of life.

The concept of devotion in this teaching helps to emphasize the importance of trust, belief, or confidence in the presence of awareness amidst the gunas' fluctuations. This trust empowers us to connect to awareness while experiencing the turbulence and change inherent to the body, mind, and life itself.

Conclusion

Lucidity, passion, dark inertia—these qualities inherent in nature bind the unchanging embodied self in the body.

(Bhagavad Gita, 14.5)[41]

He really sees who sees that all actions are performed by nature alone and that the self is not an actor.

(Bhagavad Gita, 13.29)[42]

The gunas can be understood as tools of inquiry to help us tease apart our experiences and differentiate prakriti from purusha. Before the manifestation of all phenomena, the gunas are said to be in a state of equilibrium. As the gunas move and one predominates, prakriti devolves into its many psychophysiological and environmental constituents. The gunas, in their infinitely varied proportions, create the myriad manifestations of thought, emotion, physiological state, and experience.

When we misidentify with the gunas, and thus with prakriti, we are blinded from the truth of who we are. This misperception creates suffering as we become subject to the experiences of the gunas, of agitation, inertia, and even clarity. When we understand the gunas as the substrate from which experience arises, we can see them at work. All phenomena can be broken down in this way, with the gunas as a framework for exploring thoughts, emotions, physiological states, and life occurrences. We can then begin to realize an aspect of ourselves that is wholly separate from the gunas, an observation platform from which we can witness their movement without being them. Every experience of the body, mind, and environment becomes an opportunity to distinguish prakriti from purusha and to realize unchanging awareness.

Yoga highlights that this exploration is not served by isolating from the world or shutting it out—the world assists in this journey of realization. From the foundation of the realization of unchanging awareness, we can experience the currents of delight, anger, fear, and grief while still accessing equanimity, contentment, and eudaimonic well-being.

I have seen the power of working with these ideas for people with anxiety, depression, and pain. Using the language of the gunas can shift judgment; for example, saying "rajas" instead of "fear" or "tamas" instead of "depression." Clients may be able to reflect more openly on their current experience, separate from their analysis of the "stories" that arise. Inquiry into the gunas within sensation can help people explore their thoughts, emotions, or relationship to life as they step back and notice the qualities of sattva, rajas, and tamas that constitute the experience.

Practice 3.2 Meditation: The Gunas

Let's explore the same story or situation you worked with earlier in this chapter through the lens of the gunas.

First, write out as many adjectives as you can for each of the gunas.

- Rajas: activity, creativity, motivation, agitation, anxiety, fear—anything you think of as action or mobilization.
- Sattva: clarity, illumination, lightness, joy—anything you consider part of this quality of lucidity.
- Tamas: groundedness, solidity, firmness, boundary, inertia, delusion, obscuration—anything you consider part of this quality of mass and form.

> Find a comfortable seat or lie down. Bring your attention to your breath and follow its natural rhythm.
>
> Come back to the same situation you explored earlier in this chapter (or choose to explore a different one).
>
> Release the details of the situation and your assessment of it and focus on what was, or is, experienced.
>
> - What do you notice in your body? Where do you notice it?
>   - What are the qualities of rajas, tamas, and sattva within that sensation, and how would you describe them?
> - What emotions, thoughts, or beliefs do you notice? How do you notice them? Are they also in your body? Where?
>   - What qualities of rajas, tamas, and sattva are here, and how would you describe them?
> - In this life situation itself, how do you notice the qualities of rajas, tamas, and sattva?
>
> What can you learn about the gunas that are present or dominant and how they form sensations in your body, thoughts, or the way you relate to life situations?
>
> Is there a movement, way of breathing, affirmation, or meditation that can shift this experience toward its sattvic aspects?
>
> As you strengthen the sattvic part of the experience, what would it mean to step back and find the well of sattva, or the unshakable foundation of unchanging awareness, and allow the rajas, tamas, and sattva to arise and fall? Is there a movement, affirmation, or visualization that brings you this experience?

Notes

1. Mallinson, J., & Singleton, M. (2017). *Roots of yoga*. London: Penguin.
2. Smith, J. D. (Ed.). (2009). *The Mahabharata*. London: Penguin Classics; Miller, B. S. (Trans.) (1986). *The Bhagavad-Gita: Krishna's counsel in time of war*. New York: Bantam Classics.
3. Burley, M. (2012). *Classical samkhya and yoga: An Indian metaphysics of experience*. London: Routledge; Smith, *Mahabharata*.
4. Burley, *Classical samkhya and yoga*.
5. Burley, *Classical samkhya and yoga*.
6. Miller, B. S., *Bhagavad-Gita*.
7. Miller, R. (2012). *The Samkhya Karika*. San Rafael, CA: Integrative Restoration Institute.

8. Miller, B. S., *Bhagavad-Gita*.
9. Miller, R., *Samkhya Karika*, p. 10.
10. Miller, B. S., *Bhagavad-Gita*.
11. Miller, R., *Samkhya Karika*.
12. Larson, G. J. (2014). *Classical saṃkhya: An interpretation of its history and meaning*. Delhi: Motilal Banarsidass Publishers.
13. Bawra, B. V. (2012). *Samkhya Karika*. Ravenna, OH: Brahmrishi Yoga Publications.
14. Frankl, V. E. (2006). *Man's search for meaning*. Boston, MA: Beacon Press.
15. Burley, *Classical samkhya and yoga*.
16. Miller, R., *Samkhya Karika*.
17. Burley, *Classical samkhya and yoga*.
18. Miller, R., *Samkhya Karika*.
19. Miller, B. S., *Bhagavad-Gita*.
20. Miller, B. S., *Bhagavad-Gita*.
21. Miller, B. S., *Bhagavad-Gita*.
22. Miller, B. S., *Bhagavad-Gita*.
23. Miller, B. S., *Bhagavad-Gita*.
24. Miller, B. S., *Bhagavad-Gita*.
25. Miller, B. S., *Bhagavad-Gita*.
26. Miller, B. S., *Bhagavad-Gita*.
27. Miller, B. S., *Bhagavad-Gita*.
28. Miller, B. S., *Bhagavad-Gita*.
29. Miller, B. S., *Bhagavad-Gita*.
30. Miller, B. S., *Bhagavad-Gita*.
31. Miller, B. S., *Bhagavad-Gita*.
32. Smith, *Mahabharata*.
33. Smith, *Mahabharata*.
34. Miller, B. S., *Bhagavad-Gita*.
35. Miller, B. S., *Bhagavad-Gita*.
36. Miller, B. S., *Bhagavad-Gita*.
37. Miller, B. S., *Bhagavad-Gita*.
38. Miller, B. S., *Bhagavad-Gita*.
39. Miller, B. S., *Bhagavad-Gita*.
40. Miller, B. S., *Bhagavad-Gita*.
41. Miller, B. S., *Bhagavad-Gita*.
42. Miller, B. S., *Bhagavad-Gita*.

Yoga Psychology   4
Body-Mind-Environment Relationships

How do we begin to use the experiences of the body, mind, and environment for the realization of awareness? How do we reliably differentiate the psychophysiological and environmental processes of prakriti from purusha to realize awareness?

Samkhya and Our Experience of the World

As described in Chapter 3, samkhya teaches a methodology of inquiry for exploring worldly phenomena by discerning between purusha and prakriti and recognizing the operation of the gunas. In addition to these more abstract concepts, the Samkhya Karika details the specific psychophysiological and environmental constituents of prakriti, enabling practitioners to explore their relationships to the individual components of the body, mind, and environment.

This inquiry illuminates the ways in which suffering arises and provides the path toward its alleviation. We begin to recognize that our misperception and negative relationships to the body and bodily sensation; thoughts, emotions, and beliefs; and stimuli from the environment and life situations can perpetuate suffering. By contemplating each constituent of prakriti, we learn to distinguish it from purusha. The capacity to meet phenomena with equanimity arises from this realization. Inquiry into any one part of prakriti provides clarity across the domains of body, mind, and environmental phenomena, leading to the differentiation from purusha and ultimately the realization of awareness. We begin to explore the possibility of recognizing

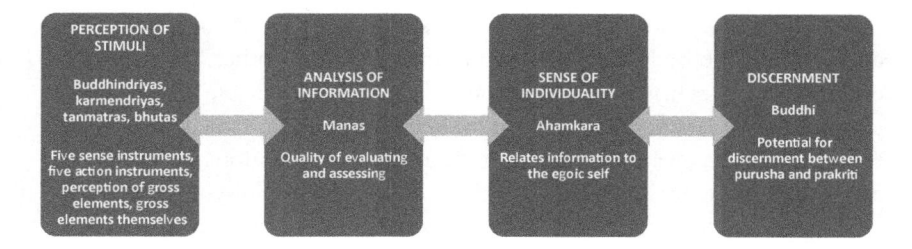

PERCEPTION OF STIMULI	ANALYSIS OF INFORMATION	SENSE OF INDIVIDUALITY	DISCERNMENT
Buddhindriyas, karmendriyas, tanmatras, bhutas	Manas	Ahamkara	Buddhi
Five sense instruments, five action instruments, perception of gross elements, gross elements themselves	Quality of evaluating and assessing	Relates information to the egoic self	Potential for discernment between purusha and prakriti

Figure 4.1 Constituents of Prakriti.

Note: Moving from left to right, the five gross elements (bhutas) make up all environmental phenomena (including our bodies). The perception of these elements *(tanmatras)*, the way we act upon and perceive the environment *(karmendriyas* and *buddhindriyas)*, is analyzed by an aspect of the mind *(manas)*. Our sense of individuality *(ahamkara)* further processes this information, including memory, needs, beliefs, and future considerations. The resulting perceptions of environmental stimuli—along with thoughts, emotions, and beliefs—are then channeled through the attribute of discernment *(buddhi)*, which allows us to discriminate between prakriti and purusha. We can then move in the other direction, from right to left in the chart, generating optimal action from this insight.

awareness within each constituent and to engage in the world from this place of equanimity, contentment, and eudaimonic well-being.

Yoga integrates these foundational samkhya teachings to offer a method that promotes contemplation and insight. When undertaken with this intention, each yogic practice assists us in examining our reactions to and relationships with what arises in the body, mind, and environment while situated in awareness.

The teachings of samkhya delineate each component of prakriti (changeable constituents of psychophysiological and environmental phenomena) from purusha (changeless observer) and from awareness. These constituents, described in Figure 4.1, are the subject of this chapter.

Buddhi: Constituent of Discernment and Wisdom

> Buddhi is discernment, its lucid (sattvika) form [comprising] dharma, knowledge, non-attachment, and masterfulness, and its darkened (tamasa) form [comprising] the opposite.
>
> (Samkhya Karika, 23)[1]

Buddhi—the "great principle" or the "intellect"—is the first constituent described as arising from prakriti. Also called discriminative wisdom, this quality holds the capacity for insight into the difference between the psychophysiological or environmental phenomena of prakriti and purusha.

Buddhi manifests in two forms: One stems from the influence of sattva and is said to be buddhi's pure or illumined form; the other, its deluded or obscured form, stems from the influence of tamas (see Table 4.1). Whether sattva or tamas is the predominant influence on buddhi affects our perception of and relationship to sensation, thoughts, and emotions as well as our actions and behavior.

When under the influence of sattva, buddhi affords us the clarity to discern purusha from prakriti, the definition of wisdom in yoga and samkhya. From this wisdom comes a healthy nonattachment to worldly phenomena. The individual exhibits a sort of mastery over the stimuli of the body, mind, and environment, meaning they experience the natural fluctuations of these three domains while remaining connected to awareness with its emergent qualities of equanimity, contentment, and eudaimonic well-being. Along with this mastery comes the capacity to understand and align with dharma so that right action can be undertaken in harmony with oneself and one's surroundings.

Table 4.1 Characteristics of Buddhi Under the Influence of Sattva and Tamas

Attribute of Awareness	Influence of Sattva	Influence of Tamas
Wisdom	Discernment between purusha and prakriti	Misperception of the difference between purusha and prakriti
Nonattachment	Healthy nonattachment to the fluctuations of body, mind, and environmental phenomena	Confusion produces unhealthy attachment to body, mind, and environmental stimuli including emotions, thoughts, beliefs, and sensations
Mastery	Ability to maintain connection to awareness amidst the fluctuations of prakriti leads to equanimity, contentment, eudaimonic well-being	Misidentification with body, mind, and environmental stimuli leads to being swept away and overwhelmed by the constant fluctuations of prakriti
Dharma	Understanding of and alignment with dharma mean that right action can be undertaken in harmony with the self and surroundings	Incapacity to see or act in alignment with dharma leads to actions that perpetuate suffering because of their disharmony with the inner and outer environment

When buddhi is under the influence of tamas, the opposite occurs: The ability to distinguish purusha from prakriti is obscured, and we "forget" our true nature as awareness. Ultimately, this misidentification with, confusion about, and unhealthy attachment to what arises in the body, mind, and environment make it difficult or impossible to take right action and suffering is perpetuated.

Whether sattva or tamas predominates determines the capacity for or accessibility of wisdom; healthy nonattachment; mastery over body, mind, and environmental stimuli; and right action in support of dharma. The characteristics of buddhi under the influence of sattva support the attributes necessary for the realization of awareness.

Clinical Relevance

Pain science is demonstrating how persistent pain results in misinterpretation of safe stimuli.[2] Any information coming into the body can be perceived as dangerous, resulting in muscular tension and fear of movement, which perpetuates the pain cycle. The patient identifies with the pain as the truth and does not perceive other possibilities, perhaps unable to notice other (nonpainful) stimuli at all or to imagine the absence of the pain. For example, evidence demonstrates that the presence of osteoarthritis alone does not necessarily correlate with the experience of pain. However, simply receiving such a diagnosis can convince a patient that osteoarthritis is causing their pain and lead to a cycle of increased disability involving fear of movement and consequently worsening tension and physical restriction.

Likewise, based on belief or past experience, someone can experience their emotions as the only possible truth. They may conceive of their anger, sadness, or fear as the only possible perspective on a situation. Attachment to a single interpretation of mental sensation can make it difficult to consider other viewpoints, diminish well-being, and damage relationships with the self and others. Ultimately, the alleviation of suffering is hindered if the person lacks the discernment to reinterpret stimuli from the body, mind, and environment.

Ahamkara: Constituent of Individuality

Ahamkara is the next constituent of prakriti given by samkhya. This term can be described as "self-shape" and includes the characteristics that define us as separate individuals. From ahamkara, the traits of egoity, self-assertion, and self-reflexive awareness arise.[3] It is important to note that although the definition of ahamkara can include egoity and the concept includes elements of ego, this yogic aspect of mind is not synonymous with ego in a psychoanalytic sense. Ahamkara represents the process of taking in information and shaping it into a sense of a separate self, a perception of individuality. This process entails forming thoughts, memories, and habits that separate what we define as our individual identity from awareness. Yogic philosophy teaches us how to become aware of other possibilities.

The attributes that emerge from ahamkara are, like buddhi, informed by the predominant influence of the gunas. Rajas, the quality of mobilization, can encourage or energize the sattvic or tamasic characteristics of this sense of individuality. As sattva is responsible for characteristics like clarity, it provides the means for "bare attention" and "mere observation" in support of the apprehension and analysis of body, mind, and environmental phenomena.[4] This illumination occurs via the mind and senses. Tama guna, in addition to being responsible for obscuration or inertia, is also the quality of form and mass; tamas brings the perception and experience of the gross and subtle elements to ahamkara.

Manas: Constituent of the "Mind"

Manas holds the capacity for synthesis, analysis, deliberation, and intentionality.[5] As the thinking aspect of the mind, manas is where information is transferred from the five senses to higher-order integration with the sense of individuality (ahamkara). It is also where information interacts with the organs of action such as the hands and feet (as described below) for engagement with the world. This constituent of prakriti is responsible for the capacity to think, evaluate, and remember. Because of these capacities, manas is said to emerge from the sattvic influence of ahamkara, providing the means for insight into the phenomena of the body, mind, and environment.

Buddhindriyas and Karmendriyas: Capacity to Sense and Act

> Sense-capacities is the term for seeing, hearing, smelling, tasting and touching; voice, hand, foot, anus and underparts are called action-capacities.
>
> (Samkhya Karika, 26)[6]

[T]he operation…of the five [sense capacities] is held to be bare awareness of sound and so forth; speaking, grasping, walking, excreting and [sexual] pleasure are [the operations of] the five [action-capacities].
(Samkhya Karika, 28)[7]

The *buddhindriyas*, sense capacities, represent the way we take in information from our surroundings. These five exteroceptive senses provide the capacity for hearing, seeing, smelling, tasting, and touching, enabling us to gain knowledge of our world. The prefix *buddhi* illumines the buddhindriyas' function of providing the perception of the outside world needed for insight and discrimination.

The *karmendriyas*, action capacities, represent the way we interact with the world and include speaking, grasping, walking, excreting, and procreating. The prefix *karm* illumines the action-producing function of these instruments.

The buddhindriyas and karmendriyas, as constituents of prakriti, enable us to perceive and experience environmental phenomena. These capacities are the doorways through which bare awareness or mere observation occur. They are simply the senses and actions themselves, without attendant judgment, categorization, or meaning.[8]

An example is useful for summarizing the relationship among prakriti's constituents. A stimulus such as sound is picked up by the ear. The buddhindriya, or capacity, of hearing brings that stimulus to the manas aspect of the mind for analysis, evaluation, and processing. Manas brings its assessment to ahamkara, where the relationship to individuality, including history, emotion, and belief, is incorporated. Ahamkara then brings this information to buddhi. Under a sattvic influence, buddhi can use all of the information to discern between purusha and prakriti—the contemplation of the sound becomes an understanding of the difference between the changing and the changeless. From this state of discriminative wisdom, buddhi can direct ahamkara, manas, and the action capacities (karmendriyas) to interact with the sound appropriately.

In short, the sequence of processing is: sound waves enter the ear ⟶ buddhindriya (process and capacity to hear) ⟶ manas ⟶ ahamkara ⟶ buddhi ⟶ karmendriya (process or capacity to act) (see Figure 4.1). In ordinary perception, this chain of events is passive, building subconsciously without our recognition or control. Yoga helps us to decide to become active participants, fully aware of the process and able to disentangle habitual response from the truth of bare awareness. When buddhi is under tamasic influence, this clarity is disrupted and the action undertaken arises from a state of misperception, confusion, and misidentification with prakriti.

Gross and Subtle Elements

From the tamasic aspect of ahamkara we experience the *tanmatras* (subtle elements or process of experiencing the gross elements) and the *bhutas* (gross elements or elements that comprise all phenomena including the body and environment).[9] The bhutas are the five elements—earth, water, fire, wind, and space—that comprise all objects of prakriti. We come into sensory contact with these elements via the tanmatras—sound, feeling, form, flavor, and odor. The tanmatras represent the way in which the objects of the world are perceived and brought to manas and ahamkara for comprehension.

Putting It Together: Understanding the Map of Exploration

Previous chapters explored a discussion in the Mahabharata in which Bhishma and Yudhisthira describe concepts such as dharma, samkhya, and yoga. This dialogue includes a metaphor to help clarify the constituents of prakriti, their functions, and their relationships with one another:

> The individual is likened to a city. Buddhi is the leader of the city, the queen. She holds the capacity for discernment and wisdom. Ahamkara and manas are the queen's advisors, responsible for collecting and conveying information to her so she can consider the action required. The sense and action capacities are the citizens, who convey information about the state of the kingdom to the advisors and who undertake action.[10]

It is important to note that each part of the process has its own unique roles and tasks. Each constituent of prakriti has specific characteristics that define its responsibilities and capacities.

- Sense and action capacities do not analyze, judge, evaluate, or determine. Rather, the buddhindriyas (sense organs) simply pass along information from the outer world to the inner gates of the city in which manas, ahamkara, and buddhi dwell. Likewise, the karmendriyas (action organs) are the conduit through which action is taken in the world—they do not distinguish or evaluate the action itself. The tanmatras, or subtle elements, are responsible for our perception of the gross elements without any judgment or evaluation—they are simply the way we perceive the elements that make up all environmental and bodily phenomena.

- The inner city is the abode of manas, ahamkara, and buddhi. These constituents, which each have specific roles, work together to take in information from the outside world (manas); relate it to individual needs, circumstances, and past and future considerations (ahamkara); and practice discrimination, ultimately to determine right action in alignment with dharma (buddhi).

In the discussion mentioned above, Bhishma tells Yudhisthira that the greatest danger to this process of discriminative wisdom—to running a city with integrity—is the overpredominance of rajas or tamas in any one of the constituents. Rajas or tamas can distort information as it is passed along. If manas or ahamkara become overwhelmed by agitation (rajas) or obscuration (tamas), they are alienated from their capacity to clearly communicate perceptions and experiences to buddhi. When this happens, the senses, or citizens, are under the sway of the unbalanced quality of the gunas and action is created from overpredominance of agitation or obscuration rather than from discernment or clarity.

Each of these categories of prakriti provide the practitioner with a focus for meditation and contemplation. Inquiry into any one constituent allows us to reflect on the ways in which we experience the phenomena of the body, mind, and environment and to cultivate discriminative wisdom for the realization of the difference between purusha and prakriti.

Practice 4.1 Meditation: Aspects of Mind (see Figure 4.1)

Sit or lie comfortably with your eyes open.

Notice what you see around you—colors, textures, and shapes. Visualize the process of color and form entering the rods and cones of the eye and being formulated into objects of identification through the manas mind. The manas aspect of the mind evaluates and assesses these shapes, forms, and categories, while the ahamkara designates a recognizable object. (For example, a furry, soft, gray shape crystallizes into *cat* instantly, before we notice what's happening.) The ahamkara also relates the input to your sense of identity—do you like or dislike what is seen? Is it comfortable or uncomfortable? How do the colors, forms, or objects relate to your sense of self and beliefs? (Cat-lover? Person with allergies or a fear of cats based on previous experience?) Buddhi teases all of this apart to distinguish the components of prakriti and to recognize that underneath all is a changeless quality, an experience of awareness from which perceptions, thoughts, and beliefs arise.

Repeat the inquiry with sound.

Close your eyes. Notice sound. Visualize sound waves hitting the eardrums and being picked up by the nerves of the ear, vibration becoming nerve impulses. Visualize how the manas aspect of the mind creates from that information recognizable categories, labels, and forms. Visualize how the ahamkara then relates this to your sense of identity. What is liked or disliked, comfortable or uncomfortable? Buddhi is the quality that allows you to notice and to step back to discern the fluctuations that are prakriti from awareness and purusha. What is it like to be situated in buddhi and to observe sensation coming into the ear, becoming a fixed object, and being related to your thoughts, emotions, and beliefs?

Repeat with an element, for example, earth.

Find a comfortable place from which to observe the element of earth. Notice how the senses pick up the element—via touch, sight, smell. Tease apart this process of the eyes taking in the color and texture, the hands taking in the feel, maybe the nose taking in the odor. Notice how manas takes information from the senses to categorize and label. What would it mean to simply see, smell, and feel without category or label? Notice how ahamkara takes in the labels from manas and creates likes and dislikes, emotions. Continue to drop beneath ahamkara's judgment and manas' labels to the color, texture, feel, and smell themselves. Can you do this without cognition? Notice buddhi watching the process of the senses taking in the earth, manas labeling, ahamkara judging. Situated in buddhi, can you be simultaneously aware of the earth itself, how the senses take it in, how manas labels, and how ahamkara judges? Can you continue to root into a noncognitive space of the earth itself, outside of all of these processes?

Causes of Enmeshment: The Lived and Habitual Bodies

Phenomenology offers a language to support the above-described exploration of our experience of the body, mind, and environment. A full discussion of phenomenology is beyond the scope of this book, but its concepts can enhance this analysis.[11]

The dynamic language of phenomenology helps to describe how the interplay of components of the body, mind, and environment create an individual's experience. Phenomenology attempts to view all phenomena with an unbiased, naïve attitude so that their essence may emerge outside habitual patterns of perception, interpretation, and interaction.[12] The experience of an individual—including thoughts, bodily perceptions or sensations, emotions, memory, and social activities—reflects a co-created trialectic between the body, mind, and environment.[13] Exploring each experience, and its meaning, can both illuminate habitual patterns of interacting with stimuli and provide insight into phenomena "as they are."[14]

Phenomenological insight has been used by healthcare professionals hoping to understand the subjective experiences of those with illness, disease, or disability.[15] This language has also been used in an explanatory model of yoga therapy, as it supports the translation of yogic concepts into research and healthcare contexts.[16] Phenomenology offers another way of understanding how relationships among the body, mind, and environment create experience (including suffering and its alleviation) and habit.

The Lived Body

The concept of the *lived body* furthers the discussion of the relationship between the body and its surrounding environment. In *Phenomenology of Perception,* Merleau-Ponty writes that "the body is the vehicle of being in the world"[17]; we must "awaken the experience of the world such as it appears to us insofar as we are in the world through our bodies, and insofar as we perceive the world with our bodies."[18] He describes this further, saying,

> One's own body is in the world just as the heart is in the organism: it continuously breathes life into the visible spectacle, animates it and nourishes it from within, and forms a system with it.[19]

The body, mind, and environment are in a continual conversation, co-creating the experience of each moment. We cannot separate the body-mind's experience from its surroundings, nor our perception of the world from the physical experience of it. The body-mind can only perceive itself through its experiences embedded in the context of the environment, and the environment comes into being in its experienced form through the perceptions of the body-mind. In the body-mind-environment trialectic, physical experience is a conduit through which we can experience suffering or its alleviation.

The individual's experience cannot be reduced to its separate components of physical, mental, and environmental stimuli; it is through their interrelationships that meaning and identity are expressed. The concept of "lived body" represents this inseparability of the body, mind, and environment in the experience of the individual. Much like purusha needs prakriti for realization and liberation, only through environmental or life experience do we come to know the world. Exploring our perception and interpretation of phenomena can lead us to understand the causes of suffering.

The yogic literature, including the Katha Upanishad and Mahabharata, uses a chariot to describe this relationship among the mind, senses, world, and the power of discrimination in the lived body. When the chariot (the body) is not being driven by a charioteer with the power of discrimination (buddhi), the horses (our senses) "run hither and thither."[20] Without the charioteer, the reins (the mind—manas and ahamkara) receive no direction, so the horses (senses) continuously chase whatever captures their attention. Without direction, the senses run toward what is pleasurable or validating to the self-identity—habitual tendencies—and away from what threatens that self-identity. The person goes wherever the senses take them and interacts with the world based on instinctual drives. This constant unchecked movement becomes the individual's lived body.

Conversely, the person can learn to access buddhi—to purposely drive the chariot rather than being pulled along by it. The person realizes that they are the "lord of the chariot" and that with a "discriminating intellect as charioteer and a trained mind as reins, they attain the supreme goal of life"[21]— uniting with awareness and transcending suffering. This capacity to direct the mind, body, and senses empowers us to act in alignment with awareness, actualizing the harmony of dharma.

The Habitual Body

The philosophy of phenomenology helps to describe the habitual tendencies involved in the relationships between the individual and the body, mind, and environment; yoga seeks to suspend these reactions. In yoga, exploring our habits is a form of inquiry that ultimately illumines the difference between purusha and prakriti and alleviates suffering that arises from these usually unexamined tendencies.

Samkhya and yoga teach that without the sattvic influence on the intellect (buddhi), we simply follow our habits of thought, emotion, belief, and relating to the world. Rather than buddhi determining the direction of the chariot (body) or controlling the reins (ahamkara and manas), the senses dictate the direction taken by the body and mind, which travel familiar terrain.

The Yoga Sutras of Patanjali teach these habitual patterns of thoughts, emotions, beliefs, bodily states, and behaviors as *samskaras,* or subliminal intentions.[22] Engaging in any one of these patterns of reaction reinforces the propensity to re-engage in them:

> Each color of action leaves memory traces corresponding to the fruition of the action.
> (Stoler-Miller, 4.8)

> When there are lapses in discrimination, distracting concepts arise from the store of subliminal impressions.
> (Stoler-Miller, 4.27)[23]

Each action of the body and world leaves a mark. When buddhi is not under sattvic control, these (usually unconscious) remembrances arise in response to stimuli and determine the direction of action and response. Each action (of body, mind, or behavior in the world) becomes the seeds that determine the next. In the absence of discernment, each past experience dictates the way we interact with the body, mind, and environment.

> Subliminal intention formed in actions…is realized in present or potential births. As long as this root exists, actions ripen into birth, a term of life, and experience in the world. These actions bear joyful or sorrowful fruits according to the actor's virtue or vice.
> (Yoga Sutras, 2.12–2.14)[24]

Merleau-Ponty considered the habitual body to be a synthesis of experience (physical and mental) in relationship to the environment, and says that "habit resides neither in thought nor in the objective body, but rather in the body as the mediator of a world."[25] Likewise, "my usual world gives rise to habitual intentions in me."[26] Habitual ways of reacting and relating to our own bodies and minds, and to the environment, are an amalgamation of how we have traversed our life experiences to that point. Each action and its result determine the way we will likely meet similar situations in the future. The habitual body's patterns of postures, thoughts, emotions, and behaviors have ensured our survival, safety, and even success. The term *habitual body* is another way of framing this concept of repeated tendencies of reactions and relationships to the world, as a well-known section from the Brihadaranyaka Upanishad teaches:

As a person acts, so he becomes in life. Those who do good become good; those who do harm become bad. Good deeds make one pure; bad deeds make one impure. You are what your deep, driving desire is. As your desire is, so is your will. As your will is, so is your deed. As your deed is, so is your destiny.

(3.4.5)[27]

The Kleshas: Forces That Obstruct Discernment

The Yoga Sutras of Patanjali describe what obscures clear sight, or the sattvic influence of buddhi, as *kleshas*. These obstacles, described below, keep us acting from habitual patterns.

1. *Avidya*—ignorance

> Ignorance is the field where the other forces of corruption develop… Ignorance is misperceiving permanence in transience, purity in impurity, pleasure in suffering, an essential self where there is no self.
>
> (Yoga Sutras, 2.4–2.5)[28]

Avidya is the primary obstacle from which the others develop. Ignorance, in this context, is the inability to discriminate between purusha and prakriti—or the misidentification with prakriti. In samkhya, this occurs when buddhi is under the influence of tama guna.

Clinical Relevance

We might see avidya in a patient who identifies as their physical condition or diagnosis, unable to open to another perspective of relating to physical stimuli. Teaching a different way to relate to sensation is crucial to the yogic process of discernment and to the alleviation of suffering. We can help this person to understand how sensations from their mind and body mix with stimuli from the world to create their present experience. Asking clients to notice the fluctuations of experience in the body, mind, and environment can help them recognize these variable experiences in each moment—and eventually their relationships to one another.

2. *Asmita*—egoism

> Egoism is the identification, as it were, of the power of the Seer (Purusha) with that of the instrument of seeing [body-mind].
> (Yoga Sutras, 2.6)[29]

Asmita results from avidya, with its misidentification with prakriti. When we have forgotten that we *are* underlying awareness within—not the psychophysiological and environmental phenomena of prakriti—we believe ourselves to be the separate identity of the body-mind and interact with phenomena from that separateness rather than from a state of connection and equanimity.

Clinical Relevance

Similar to the ideas expressed above about ahamkara, from avidya, ignorance of the difference between purusha and prakriti may lead to misidentification with the stimuli that create the separate self. A patient may begin to think they are their pain, their angst, their difficult situation. We can help the person to recognize that they are something more than this temporary, fluctuating experience, perhaps through memory or imagery of a different experience such as happiness or peace. We might help the patient to find a posture that helps them to experience something different, like strength or grounding, challenging their belief about the permanence of their current situation.

3. *Raga*—attachment to the pleasurable
4. *Dvesha*—aversion to the unpleasant

The pulls of raga and dvesha arise as we become situated in our identity as separate beings. Both raga and dvesha can help us to validate our sense of separateness, as they can help pull us toward individuality and away from the unity of awareness. This obstacle is not so much about what is positive or negative, but rather what keeps us in our separate identity and what does not.

Clinical Relevance

If a patient believes they are not strong or good enough, she will be attracted to people and situations that validate this belief (raga). We might introduce a client to the idea that she is inherently connected to all beings and can experience states of equanimity, connection, and eudaimonia. If she feels that this threatens her identity or belief system, she will be averse to such suggestions (dvesha).

Raga and dvesha are the pulls toward and away from, respectively, what fits the story of the individual as a separate self. Raga is the pull toward that which validates the story, and dvesha is the pull away from that which invalidates it. In a therapeutic context, this concept is important as we challenge clients' beliefs in their capacity to feel love, connection, peace, confidence, and strength; we will also be challenging their habits of physical, mental, and environmental interaction.

5. *Abinivesha*—fear of death or clinging to life

    As we are introduced to ideas that challenge our separate self or habitual interaction with environmental phenomena, abinivesha is the obstacle that drives us to want to keep things as they are. Habits that form our identity as separate have kept us safe and represent firmly held patterns.

Clinical Relevance

Often, patients are unsure of who they are without their pain, diagnosis, or emotional or mental habits. Fear arises around letting go of this identity. Using imagery, meditation, or postures, we can facilitate a safe yet different experience. The stronger this experience, the more the client may open to the process of change. Once he finds safety in a new way of understanding physical, mental, and environmental stimuli, he may be open to the process of inquiry and change to ease suffering.

These five kleshas, or obstacles to clear perception, influence one another. As we address one, the others are affected in the following way.

In working with abinivesha, we can help a client to let go of fear of change. If we facilitate a safe setting for transformation, she can become receptive to letting go of the patterns of reactions to the body, mind, and environment that keep her in suffering. She learns that the habits of raga and dvesha—attraction and aversion—perpetuate this pain. It becomes clear that certain activities, people, or ways of relating to the body actually perpetuate suffering. For example, her identity is tied to participating in a certain sport even if it continues to create pain, or she knows that particular people or situations are unhealthy yet continues to interact with them without boundaries. In the same way, aversions may stop her from challenging her beliefs and ultimately maintain the suffering state. For example, a fear of movement stops her from exercising, which increases tension and creates more pain.

Helping the person to identify with these pulls of attraction and aversion and their repercussions for physical and mental/emotional well-being is crucial. What was once an attraction is given boundaries and understanding; what was once an aversion is given understanding and patience. If, however, she identifies more and more strongly with these situations and pain, asmita becomes solidified. She may forget that there are other ways of relating to body, mind, or environment and consider her suffering to be permanent. We can provide clients with a remembrance of situations, or new situations, that challenge their beliefs—for example, an experience of ease or calm for someone who feels that they can never relax. This cycle ultimately stems from avidya, ignorance of one's nature as awareness—equanimity, steadfast joy, and contentment. As we help the client remember the true nature of being, her misperceptions as the separate self, unhealthy attachments to attractions and aversions, and fear of change or the collapse of individuality all diminish. This remembrance as awareness can catalyze the process through which suffering eases.

Conclusion

The philosophy of samkhya describes how our perceptions and interpretations of the environment, mind (thoughts, emotions, beliefs), and body color our interactions with these phenomena. Without the sattvic influence on buddhi, our relationships with environmental phenomena are driven by our senses and habits. These habits then create the next moment in a continual cycle of action and reaction.

Patterns of physical, emotional, and behavioral relationships develop between what we perceive in the world and within ourselves and these phenomena. In this way, belief and habit inform our thoughts, emotions, and behavior. As Miller's translation of the Samkhya Karika states,

> By engaging in emotions, beliefs, and actions that tend toward vice we descend into misperception and delusion that lead to bondage and suffering. By engaging in emotions, beliefs, and actions that tend toward virtue we ascend into higher orders of understanding that lead to liberation.
>
> (44)[30]

We can develop ways of relating to the body, mind, and environment that cultivate the sattvic influence on buddhi. Buddhi then becomes the charioteer skillfully maneuvering action in the world; navigating the fluctuations of the body, mind, and world; and directing us toward the realization of awareness.

We can choose in any moment to connect to those emotions, beliefs, and actions that reinforce habitual patterns that lead to suffering. Conversely, we can foster new patterns that align us with dharma, virtue, and ultimately the alleviation of suffering. Within the constituent of buddhi lies a possible spectrum from wisdom to misperception; from healthy nonattachment to misidentification with environmental phenomena; from mastery to becoming overpowered by the fluctuations of prakriti; from the capacity to act in alignment with dharma to action that antagonizes it. The kinds of action that come from buddhi are determined by the influence of sattva or tamas and are said to be both innately present and capable of being developed through life experience.

The Samkhya Karika teaches that only the inner instruments (buddhi, ahamkara, and manas) hold the capacity for consideration, determination, and judgment. The senses and action capacities, in contrast, do not analyze the environmental stimuli with which they interact. Furthermore, only the inner instrument has the capacity to reflect on past experience and future considerations. Subliminal intentions, habits, or patterns—samskaras—reside only in the inner instruments, not the outer sense and action capacities and subtle or gross elements.

The concepts of lived and habitual body are significant to yoga's therapeutic application, as what is happening objectively in a client's body often differs from their subjective experience. Yoga therapy works with this subjective experience to help clients move toward equanimity, eudaimonic well-being, and a reorientation to pain, illness, or disability. This will be further explained in Chapter 6.

Notes

1. Burley, M. (2012). *Classical samkhya and yoga: An Indian metaphysics of experience*. London: Routledge.
2. For more information on this idea see the work of Lorimer Moseley and David Butler; for example, Butler, D. S., & Moseley, G. L. (2013). *Explain pain* (2nd ed.). Adelaide City West: Noigroup Publications. See also, Pearson N., Prosko, S., & Sullivan, M. (Eds.). (2019). *Yoga and science in pain care: Treating the person in pain*. London: Singing Dragon.
3. Burley, *Classical samkhya and yoga*; Miller, R. (2012). *The Samkhya Karika*. San Rafael, CA: Integrative Restoration Institute.
4. Miller, *Samkhya Karika*.
5. Burley, *Classical samkhya and yoga*; Miller, *Samkhya Karika*.

6. Burley, *Classical samkhya and yoga.*
7. Burley, *Classical samkhya and yoga.*
8. Burley, *Classical samkhya and yoga*; Miller, *Samkhya Karika.*
9. Burley, *Classical samkhya and yoga*; Miller, *Samkhya Karika.*
10. Adapted from Smith, J. D. (Ed.). (2009). *The Mahabharata.* London: Penguin.
11. For an in-depth exploration of the relationship between phenomenology and Samkhya, see Burley *Classical samkhya and yoga.*
12. Dowling, M. (2007). From Husserl to van Manen. A review of different phenomenological approaches. *International Journal of Nursing Studies, 44*(1), 131–142; Martin, J., Sugarman, J., & Slaney, K. L. (Eds.). (2015). *The Wiley handbook of theoretical and philosophical psychology: Methods, approaches, and new directions for social sciences.* Hoboken, NJ: Wiley-Blackwell.
13. Fusar-Poli, P., & Stanghellini, G. (2009). Maurice Merleau-Ponty and the "Embodied Subjectivity" (1908–61). *Medical Anthropology Quarterly, 23*(2), 91–93; Moya, P. (2014). Habit and embodiment in Merleau-Ponty. *Frontiers in Human Neuroscience, 8.* https://doi.org/10.3389/fnhum.2014.00542
14. Dowling, From Husserl to van Manen; Carel, H. (2011). Phenomenology and its application in medicine. *Theoretical Medicine and Bioethics, 32*(1), 33–46; Edwards, I., Jones, M., Thacker, M., & Swisher, L. L. (2014). The moral experience of the patient with chronic pain: Bridging the gap between first and third person ethics. *Pain Medicine, 15*(3), 364–378; Greenfield, B. H., & Jensen, G. M. (2010). Understanding the lived experiences of patients: Application of a phenomenological approach to ethics. *Physical Therapy, 90*(8), 1185–1197.
15. Carel, Phenomenology and its application in medicine; Edwards, Jones, Thacker, & Swisher, The moral experience of the patient with chronic pain; Greenfield & Jensen, Understanding the lived experiences of patients.
16. Sullivan, M. B., Moonaz, S., Weber, K., Taylor, J. N., & Schmalzl, L. (2018). Toward an explanatory framework for yoga therapy informed by philosophical and ethical perspectives. *Alternative Therapies in Health and Medicine, 24,* 38–47.
17. Merleau-Ponty M. (2012). *Phenomenology of perception* (D. A. Landes, Trans.), p. 84. New York, NY: Routledge.
18. Merleau-Ponty, *Phenomenology of perception,* p. 210.
19. Merleau-Ponty, *Phenomenology of perception,* p. 209.
20. *The Upanishads* (Vol. 2), translated by Eknath Easwaran, founder of the Blue Mountain Center of Meditation, copyright 1987, 2007; reprinted by permission of Nilgiri Press, P. O. Box 256, Tomales, CA 94971, www.bmcm.org.
21. Easwaran, *The Upanishads,* pp. 81–82.
22. Stoler-Miller, B. (1998). *Yoga: Discipline of freedom.* New York: Bantam Books.
23. Stoler-Miller, *Yoga.*
24. Stoler-Miller, *Yoga.*
25. Merleau-Ponty, *Phenomenology of perception,* p. 146.
26. Merleau-Ponty, *Phenomenology of perception,* p. 84.
27. Easwaran, *The Upanishads.*
28. Stoler-Miller, *Yoga.*
29. Satchidananda. (1990). *The Yoga Sutras of Patanjali.* Yogaville, VA: Integral Yoga Publications.
30. Miller, *Samkhya Karika.*

The Subtle Body   5
Exploring Tantra and Prana

> One beautiful spring day, the Pandavas and their friends joined together to enjoy a relaxing picnic. Arjuna and Krishna separated from the group to have a private conversation. As they talked, a tall, withered figure in a hood and cloak of rags approached. They could see that his beard and hair were yellow-orange and matted, his yellowed eyes blazing with intensity. Arjuna and Krishna stood up as this man walked toward them. The man said he was in dire need of assistance and wanted their help. Arjuna and Krishna agreed to help to the best of their ability and asked what they could do.
>
> The man took off his hood to reveal a flaming red head of hair and introduced himself as the god of fire: "I am Agni," he said. He continued:
>
> > I have been poisoned by a king who wanted to perform the grandest of ceremonies—the magnitude of which had never been accomplished by anyone. To achieve his monumental goal, the king fed me ghee for 12 years straight. This caused me to lose my color, strength, and energy, and I can no longer burn or shine.
> >
> > I went to Brahman to ask how to regain my strength. Brahman said I must eat the medicinal herbs of the Khandava Forest, the only thing that will heal my sickness. I went to the forest and tried many times to consume it. However, each time I began to ignite the trees, Indra, the king of the gods, would rain down and extinguish my flame. Indra's friend, the king of the serpents, lives in the Khandava Forest, and Indra is protecting this friend. Even though many of the

creatures inside the forest have become the enemies of the gods, they are protected from my fire because of Indra's protection of his friend.

I went back to Brahman and told him about Indra thwarting my ability to heal. He said to seek you two—that you would be able to help me to consume the forest, to return to my nature. You could also prevent these creatures of the forest, the gods' enemies, from escaping.

Arjuna and Krishna agreed to help but said they needed the right weapons. Arjuna told Agni that he needed a strong bow and a quiver of inexhaustible arrows. Krishna said he needed a chariot that was strong and as fast as the wind. Agni sought these out and provided a suitable chariot and a famous bow with a limitless supply of arrows.

Arjuna, Krishna, and Agni approached the Khandava Forest. Agni began to consume the forest, setting it alight while Krishna and Arjuna circled around it. They built a tent of arrows over the forest to shield Agni's fire from any rain that Indra might bring down to extinguish the flames. Krishna and Arjuna worked to both create this shield and prevent any creature from escaping the forest. With this protection, Agni's fire was able to gain strength and began to consume the forest.

Indra was alerted to the burning of the forest and went to protect his friend and extinguish the flames of Agni. Indra threw down torrents of rain, but his force was no match for Krishna and Arjuna's protection.

Ultimately, Agni was able to consume the forest and thus regain his vitality and nature. After the forest had been reduced to ashes, Indra presented himself to Agni, Arjuna, and Krishna. Indra, who we learn is Arjuna's father, tells his son he is proud that he was able to accomplish a feat that a celestial (Agni) could not. Indra offers a boon to both Arjuna and Krishna. Arjuna asks for all of Indra's weapons to fight a great battle to come, while Krishna asks for Arjuna's eternal friendship.

Adapted from translations by K. Ganguli, J. D. Smith, and K. Dharma[1]

Before we explore the meaning of this story and dive into its symbolism, we must define several additional components of yoga philosophy. Whereas samkhya is a dualist philosophy in which prakriti is considered separate from purusha, tantra offers a nondual perspective. In samkhya, liberation from suffering involves cultivating discrimination between the elements, capacity to sense and act upon the environment, aspects of the mind and ego, and ultimately discrimination between purusha and prakriti. Through samkhya's practices, we learn to identify the obstacles to the realization of awareness and to disentangle from misidentification with prakriti—or psychophysiological and environmental phenomena.

Seen through tantra's nondual perspective, purusha and prakriti are not separate entities. The body-mind-environment awareness relationship is a unitive, dynamic process of nonseparation. This perspective emphasizes that physical experience is a path toward liberation rather than a hindrance. The body becomes an "inner universe," a microcosm of the macrocosm, and a mechanism through which to realize awareness and alleviate suffering. This chapter explores this appreciation and investigation of the body and materiality through the concept of the subtle body. Building on our previous discussion, we will consider the *koshas, chakras, granthis,* and *prana* to help define the subtle body, then return to the story of the Khandava Forest to consider its importance to yoga therapy.

Understanding the Subtle Body: The Koshas

Kosha, often defined as "sheath," describes the constituents of the human experience from the grossest levels of the physical body to gradually more subtle levels of "vital energy," mind, and awareness.[2] Although there are many different descriptions and layers depending on the tradition and text, the model offered by the Taittiriya Upanishad is often used[3] (see Figure 5.1).

Annamaya, the Physical Sheath

Annamaya is the physical body and all of its systems—cardiovascular, respiratory, digestive, musculoskeletal, and so on. This is the layer of gross materiality of the human body.

Pranamaya, the Vital Sheath

Pranamaya is the breath itself, as well as energy, vitality, or life force. The Upanishads describe pranamaya—and the remaining three sheaths—as contained within the physical sheath.

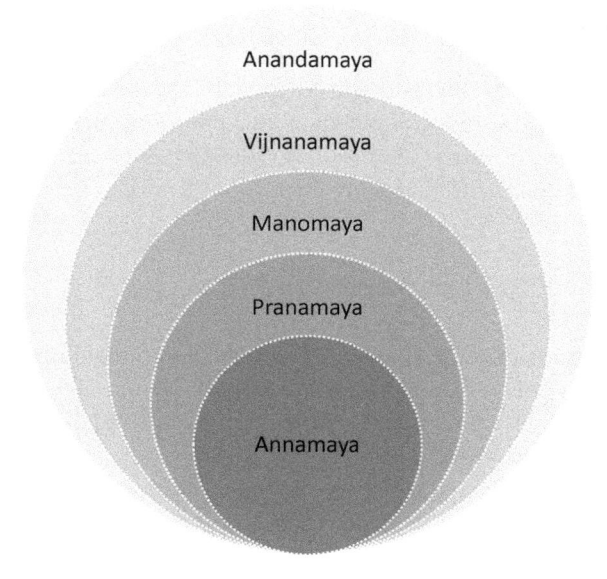

Figure 5.1 A Common Way of Depicting the Koshas, in Which One Sheath Is Encircled by the Next.

Note: The layers move from grossest in the innermost circle to most subtle in the outermost, but each layer influences the others.

The idea of an energy body can be a difficult, esoteric concept for clients to grasp, and I have found the following useful in explaining its significance. All of the systems of our bodies contribute to our level of vitality, or energy. When the cardiorespiratory system is working optimally all of the body's tissues are oxygenated effectively, enhancing our vitality, or the amount of energy we have at our disposal. Similarly, when the gastrointestinal system is working optimally we absorb nutrients effectively, when the endocrine system is working well our hormone levels are balanced and regulated, and when the nervous system is working well we can sense the internal and external environment to assess what is arising and respond appropriately. Well-running systems enhance our sense of clarity and vitality and afford us access to deeper energetic reserves.

The subtle sheath of pranamaya can be understood as the felt expression of the body systems' functioning. When annamaya—our physical systems—functions optimally our energy and vitality are optimal. Likewise, when our energy or vitality is optimal annamaya functions optimally.

Manomaya, the Mental Sheath

This sheath refers to the concepts of manas and ahamkara explored in Chapter 4. *Manomaya* includes our thoughts, emotions, beliefs, and sense of individuality. As previously discussed, misidentification with this sheath can lead to or perpetuate suffering as we forget our identity as awareness.

Vijnanamaya, the Wisdom Sheath

The sheath of *vijnanamaya* shares similar qualities to buddhi, including discriminative wisdom. Vijnanamaya is composed of faith (or trust), righteousness (or virtue, honesty, or justice), truth, meditation, and detachment.[4] This list helps us to discern what is meant by *wisdom,* as distinct from concepts such as knowledge or intelligence, in the yogic tradition.

The Taittiriya Upanishad's description illustrates that wisdom is cultivated through meditation, detachment, and trust. Without healthy detachment, we can overidentify with the phenomena of the body, mind, and environment. Without trust and faith, we can become overwhelmed by life's situations. Together, healthy detachment and trust empower us to explore the ever-changing phenomena of prakriti without becoming overwhelmed by them.

Truth and righteousness are also described as important to the development of wisdom. These qualities become the instruments with which we meet what arises in the body, mind, and environment. The capacity and willingness to meet all of life's circumstances with an inquiry into the truth of the present moment enables discrimination between fluctuating prakriti and awareness. This realization of truth provides the freedom to take right action in alignment with virtue, honesty, and justice.

Anandamaya, the Bliss Sheath

The Taittiriya Upanishad describes *anandamaya* as composed of joy, contentment, delight, and Brahman.[5] In this layer of experience, we begin to realize ourselves as awareness. With its transformative potential, defining anandamaya simply as "bliss" may diminish our understanding of this sheath. Diane Finlayson, chair of the yoga therapy program at Maryland University of Integrative Health describes this layer as "connecting to Awe," given its ability to connect us to the whole of consciousness.[6]

Diving into our subtle experiences, beyond the body, energy, mind, and wisdom, we find the possibility to realize ourselves as awareness. As mentioned in the Taittiriya Upanishad and reiterated in previous chapters, when we connect to and remember our essential nature as awareness, qualities like contentment and steadfast joy emerge.

The Kosha Model to Illuminate Relationships Among Body, Energy, and Mind

The kosha model offers a holistic way to investigate the relationships among the layers of our experience, from the gross to the subtle. Each sheath is influenced by the others—what arises in one affects all. This tantric view does not consider the mind and body as separate entities, but rather as a continuum of experience. As Christopher Wallis says, "The mind is the subtlest aspect of body, and the body the most tangible manifestation of the mind."[7]

The three grosser layers of annamaya (physical phenomena), pranamaya (energetic experience), and manomaya (mental experience) can become entry points for analyzing our experiences and cultivating insight. We can use this model to explore how our habitual ways of relating to and reacting to all stimuli are due to the interaction of these three layers of body, energy, and mind (see Figure 5.2).

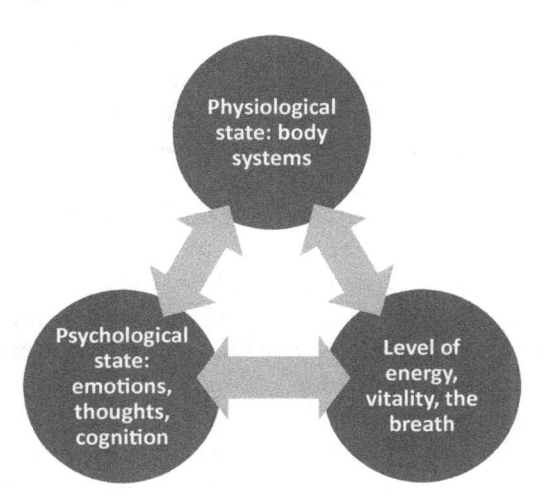

Figure 5.2 Cycle of Concurrent Influences Among Body, Energy, and Mind in the Creation of Present-Moment Experience.

Note: In our daily, habitual interactions with phenomena, we filter experiences through the reactions of our physical, energetic, and psychoemotional states.

Although what happens in each kosha occurs concurrently, we can use this model to tease apart the layers of experience and investigate what is arising in each layer of the body, energy, and mind separately while exploring the reciprocal effects. Separating what is happening in each kosha may not accurately represent the full human experience, but it does provide a useful way to examine each layer for greater insight as well as discernment to address fundamental concerns. As Finlayson says, we can use this model to begin work with clients in the area where they are most conscious of discomfort.[8]

We can consider a sympathetically activated system (fight or flight response) as initiated through the portals of the body, energy, or mind.

- **Portal of annamaya.** *Whatever arises in the physical body affects the experience of energy, or vitality, as well as thoughts and emotions.*
  When the sympathetic response is activated in annamaya, changes are reflected in both pranamaya and manomaya. In pranamaya, we might observe faster, often dysfunctional or shallow breathing patterns and heightened or agitated energy levels. In manomaya, this activation can take the form of a range of emotional and cognitive responses, from excitement or anger to anxiety, as well as negative appraisal of situations or rumination.
- **Portal of pranamaya.** *A change in the level of energy, vitality, or breath affects physiological systems as well as thoughts and emotions.*
  This same cascade of events can start with pranamaya. Dysfunctional breathing patterns (e.g., shallow or fast breathing) or a feeling of agitated, heightened energy can lead to the same physiological activation of the sympathetic nervous system in annamaya kosha, and cognitive/emotional activations in manomaya.
- **Portal of manomaya.** *What arises in the mind also affects breath patterns, energy levels, and physiological activations.*
  Starting from manomaya, anxious or worried thoughts can lead to an agitation of energy or altered breathing patterns and the activation of physiological systems involved in the sympathetically driven fight-or-flight state in pranamaya and annamaya, respectively.

The kosha model provides insight into how each layer of experience is inextricably linked to the others. By affecting one, we affect the others. From a therapeutic perspective, we can utilize any of these layers of body, energy, or mind to develop an understanding of habitual patterns that may cause suffering. The model helps us to work with one layer of experience as a catalyst for change in the others.

Changing Habits of Relationship: Through the Lens of Vijnanamaya and Anandamaya

I often describe the more subtle sheaths of vijnanamaya and anandamaya as structures that can help change habitual reactions to what arises in the grosser layers of annamaya, pranamaya, and manomaya (see Figure 5.3).

Vijnanamaya is described above as the sheath of wisdom. Some models also explain that beliefs are a more subtle aspect of vijnanamaya that influences our emotions, thoughts, energy, and physical patterns. As the sheath through which wisdom emerges, vijnanamaya kosha enables insight into the phenomena of the three grosser koshas. Through its intrinsic qualities of truth, trust, healthy detachment, and virtue, we can disentangle from habitual reactions to physiological, energetic, and emotional experiences—including long-held patterns of

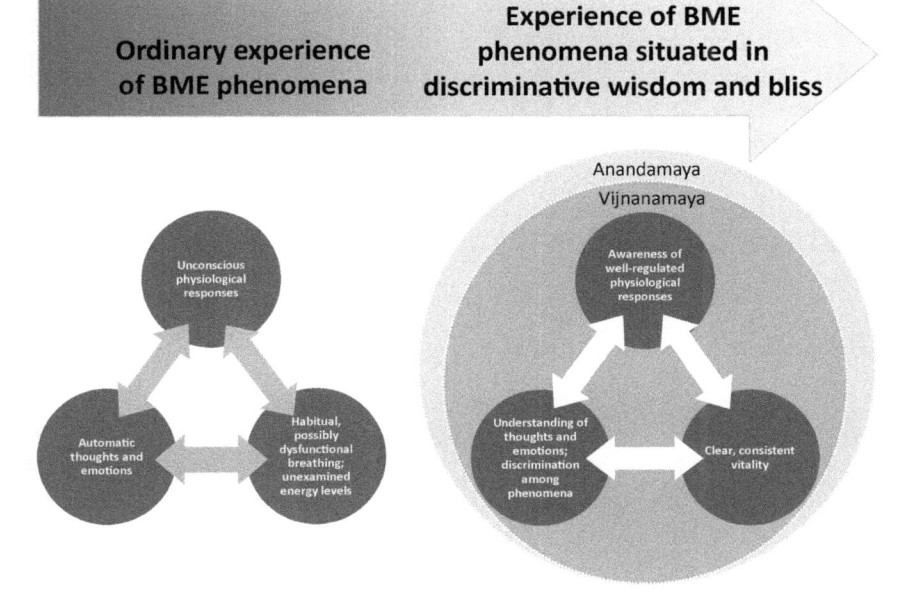

Figure 5.3 Shifting Our Experience of the Body, Mind, and Environment From Habit to Insight.

Note: Through the lens of anandamaya and vijnanamaya, yoga can help us shift our relationship with the phenomena of the body, mind, and environment (BME) from habitual response to insight. These subtle koshas ultimately enable a connection to unwavering contentment amid fluctuating phenomena. Wisdom and bliss then color all of our daily interactions so we can act in new ways that mitigate suffering.

belief. The wisdom of vijnanamaya enables both discernment between and insight into the relationships occurring in the phenomena of the body, energy, and mind. Ultimately, the wisdom sheath enables differentiation of the more gross levels of experience from awareness.

An example of vijnanamaya at work is when clients begin to understand how they hold stress or tension in their bodies. Once they learn what tightness feels like in their muscles, they often have the insight that every time they become stressed or overwhelmed, the tension in their hip flexors, jaw, or lower back returns. The person learns to identify patterns of how stress or overwhelm in the mind are reflected by tightness in their muscles. This musculoskeletal tension can then become a signal through which the person recognizes their mental stressors and an indication to do something for its alleviation—movement, a breath practice, an evaluation of life needs.

Anandamaya, composed of unwavering joy or steady contentment can also shift the person's relationship with body, mind, and environmental phenomena. The person can learn to perceive what is arising in the grosser three layers—for example, discomfort in annamaya, lethargy in pranamaya, or sadness in manomaya—and still recognize awareness, through which steady contentment and equanimity may emerge. Understanding our true essence as awareness enables us to meet each phenomenon differently, from a place of joy and delight. Clients in pain develop the ability to experience their pain alongside their joy, their sadness alongside their contentment, their agitation alongside their equanimity.

The Subtle Body Detailed

Exploring Pranamaya

The koshas provide an overall picture of complex layers of experience on a continuum from the gross to subtle and their interconnections. Chapter 4 breaks down manomaya to enable exploration of the various aspects of the mind, including manas as the thinking, categorizing, labeling component, and ahamkara as the sense of "I" and seat of emotional responses to stimuli. Here, we focus on pranamaya as a subtle bridge between the body and mind.

The layer of pranamaya serves as a two-way conduit through which physical and psychological processes influence and are reflected in one another. Through this sheath, what arises in the body is reflected in the mind, just as what arises in the mind is reflected in the body. Situated between the physical and mental/emotional layers of experience, pranamaya can be an entry point for examination as well as a link between physiological and psychological processes. In other words, the level of energy we experience influences and is influenced by myriad processes related to nourishment, environment, interpersonal relationships, sleep, body-system function, thoughts, mood, emotions, and so on.

In his 2012 book *Tantra Illuminated*, Christopher Wallis describes this layer of vital energy or life force as

> the interface between the physical body and the mind...though it is subtler and more fundamental than either. It is, in a sense, the *means* by which the mind extends itself throughout the body in the form of what is called the "subtle body."[9]

This subtle body of pranamaya has been described in various ways throughout yogic tradition. For our exploration, we will first consider prana and the prana vayus, followed by subtle body maps such as the chakras and granthis.

Prana and the Prana Vayus

Prana is the life breath, the vital energy that animates all living things.[10] Yogic texts like the Upanishads, Samkhya Karika, and Mahabharata describe five directions, forms, or functions of this vital energy—the *prana vayus*.[11] The prana vayus circulate and energize the entire human body-mind system.

These five functions of prana are present in the body as well as in the mental faculties including manas, ahamkara, and buddhi. Our thinking, emotions, sense of individuality, and capacity for discrimination are influenced and supported by these five currents of vital energy. Each prana vayu is said to have a particular directional flow and location in the body.[12]

The following descriptions of the five vayus and their functions (see Table 5.1) are influenced by the teachings of Richard Miller and Sandra Anderson, as well as the aforementioned yogic texts.

Prana Vayu

- Location: This vital energy is said to reside in the nose, mouth, heart, lungs, chest, and head.
- Function: Prana vayu is responsible for receiving information or stimuli. This can include the inspiration of breath, as well as taking in ideas, concepts, and perspectives, along with sensitivity to inner or outer sensations/stimuli.

Table 5.1 Summary of the Prana Vayus

Vayu	Attribute	Location
Prana	Capacity to receive, take in, sense (both inner and outer perceptions, sensations)	Heart/lungs
Apana	Capacity to let go, release, including releasing of habits, thoughts, behaviors	Pelvis
Samana	Capacity to integrate and assimilate information	Navel
Udana	Capacity to articulate; self-expression	Throat
Vyana	Capacity for change, expansion, fluidity	Throughout the body, limbs

- Examples of healthy prana vayu include being aware of inner bodily sensations, feelings, and emotions and an ability to receive.
- An imbalance in prana vayu can manifest in an inability to receive experiences like joy, love, kindness, and compassion or inability to perceive inner bodily sensation or emotions.

Apana Vayu

- Location: This vital energy is said to reside in the pelvis, lower abdomen, lower body, and back of the body.
- Function: Apana vayu is responsible for elimination, letting go, and the outward flow of information. This can include the exhalation of breath as well as release of ideas, emotional states, and physical tension.
- Examples of healthy apana vayu include being able to relax, experiencing a calm mind, and letting go of unhealthy physical, mental, or behavioral habits.
- An imbalance in apana vayu may include an inability to release unhealthy attachment to negative states like fear, worry, doubt, anger, or confusion.

Samana Vayu

- Location: This vital energy is said to reside in the navel and central area of the body.
- Function: Samana vayu is responsible for assimilation and digestion, including physical as well as sensory perceptions, thoughts, emotions, feelings, and ideas. This vital energy is often depicted as flowing in a spiral from the periphery to the core of the body.

- Examples of healthy samana vayu include the integration of the energies of prana and apana vayu. The movement of samana vayu reflects the capacity to let go to make space for new perceptions and insight.
- An imbalance in samana vayu might be seen when a person remains stuck in habitual reactions and relationships to body, mind, and environmental phenomena. They may begin to realize what needs to be brought in and released but are unable to move into a new way of relating to arising phenomena and instead remain in cycles of suffering. In contrast, a person with healthy samana vayu would be aware of what needs to be brought in (e.g., confidence, vitality, compassion), could identify any resistance or what needs to be released (e.g., anger, hurt, low self-esteem), and is willing to explore what needs to happen to effect change. Inquiry into alternative perspectives, feelings, and physical sensations enables new possibilities for relating to arising phenomena.

Udana Vayu

- Location: This vital energy is said to reside in the throat and upper palate.
- Function: Udana vayu is responsible for upward movement of energy, speech, and expression, and for the capacity to articulate.
- Healthy udana vayu enables articulation of feelings, emotions, or ideas.
- An imbalance in udana vayu is reflected in an inability to articulate what arises in physical, energetic, or mental experience; this would include inability to articulate what needs to be brought in (prana vayu), what needs to be released (apana vayu), and what new relationships need to develop (samana vayu).

Vyana Vayu

- Location: This vital energy is said to reside throughout the entire body.
- Function: Vyana vayu is responsible for circulation and expansion, including the integration and coordination of the other vayus and movement of vital energy throughout the system. Often pictured in a circular flow, vyana vayu is samana vayu's counterpart as it spreads outward from the core. Vyana vayu represents the capacity to take in information via prana vayu, let go what is no longer needed via apana vayu, integrate change processes via samana vayu, articulate that movement via udana vayu, and ultimately change when needed. This vayu represents the capacity to move from mere insight into engaged action to create new patterns that lead to the alleviation of suffering.

- Examples of healthy vyana vayu include the capacity to be fluid and readiness for change. This vayu represents the stage at which a person is ready to take on new perspectives.
- An imbalance in vyana vayu would be seen in situations where the person is not ready to adopt new perspectives or to change their relationships with body, mind, and environmental phenomena.

> **Practice 5.1 Short Reflection: The Prana Vayus**
>
> Sit for a moment in quiet contemplation.
> - *Prana vayu*: Consider what you need to allow in and receive. To experience relaxation, ease, comfort, love, connection?
> - *Apana vayu*: What needs to be let go so that you can receive this intention? Anger, hurt, resentment, feeling of not deserving?
> - *Samana vayu*: Contemplate the experience of allowing what needs to be brought in and what needs to be let go. What new experience, thought, or affirmation emerges? Confidence, acceptance, contentment?
> - *Udana vayu*: How would you articulate this new experience that needs to arise to allow what is needed and release what needs to be let go? Is there an image, affirmation?
> - *Vyana vayu*: Find this new experience within the body and mind. Is there a way of standing or moving that helps you embody this fully? What kinds of thoughts, emotions, and ways of relating to others would emerge from this?

Nadis, Chakras, and Granthis: Subtle-Body Maps

Whereas prana is the vital energy that flows through the body and the five prana vayus are directions and functions of that energy, yogic teachings also include specific maps of the subtle body these energies inhabit. These maps illustrate how energy flows through the system as well as potential places of obstruction. Although the texts and teachings of yoga contain many variations on subtle-body maps, we can draw themes from their commonalities. Most of the discussion below follows Mallinson and Singleton's synthesis.[13]

Prana flows through the subtle body within a network of channels, or *nadis*, often said to number 72,000.[14] The yogi is taught to direct vital energy from these more peripheral nadis to a central channel, *sushumna*, whereby it is drawn upward through the subtle body. Yogic practices such as asana, pranayama, mudras, certain meditations, and visualizations are intended to stimulate prana and direct it into sushumna. The ascent and unobstructed movement of prana symbolizes a path to liberation from suffering.

When prana rises through sushumna, it moves from the base of the pelvis through the crown of the head. Along this central path lie energetic structures called *chakras* and *granthis*. Chakras can be defined as wheels or vortices, and granthis as knots. These "structures" symbolize places along the path of sushumna where prana's vital energy can become stuck or blocked. When the chakras or granthis block the flow of prana, they become obstacles on the yogi's journey toward liberation.

The number and meaning of the chakras vary with text, tradition, and culture. Some traditions teach the chakras as already present within the subtle body, whereas others teach that the yogi creates them through meditation and visualizations. Either way, these subtle energy structures become objects of meditation through which to both notice obstructions to the flow of prana and to discover ways to facilitate its free passage through them.

The granthi model offers another way of representing the obstacles to prana's ascent. As knots along the central channel, granthis can entangle prana and therefore obstruct its flow. The three main granthis are at the pelvis, abdomen, and throat, common places where prana can become blocked. When these knots are pierced prana can continue its rise along sushumna.[15]

Yogis use the subtle-body models of the nadis, chakras, and granthis to both visualize and manipulate prana. The various yoga practices activate prana, move it from the periphery to sushumna, and enable it to pierce through the granthis and chakras for ascent and liberation.

A Brief Foray Into Tantra

Tantric teachings expound on these subtle-body ideas. The word *tantra* has many meanings and refers to both a body of texts and the practices and knowledge found within them.[16] The root *tan*—to propagate, extend, stretch, elaborate, expand upon—combines with *tra*—to save or protect.[17] Wallis thus defines the concept as, "Tantra spreads (tan) wisdom that saves (tra)."[18]

Richard Miller teaches that tantra helps us to understand the unity of our true nature, "where we stand free of psychological, cultural and philosophical conditioning in the truth of what actually is. We discover we are a vastness that is infinite, joyous, loving, kind, compassionate and always present even in the midst of difficulty."[19] The koshas describe the ways in which we are embodied as unique human beings, but we are more than these five sheaths. Tantra reveals that which is beyond the body, mind, senses, and the observer as a separate entity.[20]

Common tantric themes include the following.

- Tantra is a nondual tradition. It evolves and elaborates upon the practices found within samkhya and the Yoga Sutras of Patanjali and includes meditation, pranayama, asana, mantra, mandala, ritual, and activation of subtle energy centers. Much of today's body-based hatha yoga derives from this tantric perspective and integrates teachings from the Yoga Sutras and samkhya.[21]
- Tantra emphasizes experiential practices, rather than intellectual or cognitive processes, to explore the body, mind, and environment and to realize one's true nature as awareness.[22]
- Tantra is often differentiated by its focus on energy or power, with special attention given to the empowerment of the body.[23]
  - "As above, so below" is often used to describe this concept of the individual as a microcosm of the universal macrocosm. External phenomena are mirrored in the individual's inner experience to become symbols for reflection and insight. Entire inner worlds comprise heavens, hells, mountains, forests, and oceans.[24] Forests represent internal places that may be obscured, unclear, or unknown; mountains signify places of strength, groundedness, and stability; and oceans symbolize places of fluidity and dynamism.
  - A powerful teaching describes our experiences as various worlds that we create, inhabit, and become. There is a whole world that is anger. This world includes specific postures, muscular tensions, physical sensations, thoughts, emotions, beliefs, and even ways of perceiving and interacting with others and the external world. The same could be said about the worlds of happiness, grief, gratitude, and so on—each carries its own set of physical, mental, emotional, and behavioral attributes.

Empowerment of the Body: Entextualization and Svadhyaya

In his 2005 book, *The Tantric Body: The Secret Tradition of Hindu Religion,* Gavin Flood uses the term *entextualization* to describe how the yogi's body becomes inscribed and mapped onto by the texts and teachings of tantra.[25] In entextualization, the body serves as the metaphor and medium through which the teachings are internalized into lived experience.[26] The body becomes the representation of the teachings through which realization occurs.

Tantra moves away from interpretation or intellectual endeavors to elucidate the importance of internalizing the teachings for this embodied realization.[27] The embodied experience is recognized as essential to the process of inquiry that leads to the realization of awareness and the alleviation of suffering. As Flood writes, the text becomes "expressed as body and the body articulated in the text."[28]

Yoga therapist and professor Amy Wheeler teaches that the word *svadhyaya*, a niyama in Patanjali's Yoga Sutras, shares this idea of entextualization. *Sva* signifies self, *dhy* signifies the yogic limb of absorption, and *ya* signifies texts. Svadhyaya can thus be understood as absorption of the self within the texts, or "self-text."

Entextualization happens through years of dedicated effort, disciplined practice, and deep study. The process entails reading the texts and visualizing their teachings within the individual's inner experience using practices such as ritual, meditation, asana, and mudra.[29] Discovery of the tantric body occurs as the energetic structures—nadis, chakras, and granthis—are mapped onto the individual.

This focus on experiencing the teachings rather than intellectualizing the principles empowers us with the capacity to enact the lessons in life situations. Tantra is thus very much a fluid, living tradition that evolves with time and culture—it is philosophy in action.

The Body-Mind-Environment as Guide

The teachings of tantra help to diminish the misconception that the body, mind, and environment are separate from awareness; all phenomena must be explored and are part of awareness. Rather than disengaging from physical, mental/emotional, or worldly experiences, these become part of the path, and the practitioner understands the psychophysiological materiality of prakriti as not separate from awareness. Everything arising from the body, mind, and environment is an aspect of awareness and thus a guide along the path of realization.

We can look to the elements of earth, water, fire, and so on, as well as to our own bodies or minds, to help us realize awareness. As we come to understand these phenomena, we understand awareness. In the meditations that follow, which I learned from Richard Miller, you might choose to work with one of the elements at a time (Practices 5.2–5.6), or consider each in turn during a single session.

Practice 5.2 Body, Mind, and Environment Reflecting Awareness—Earth

Go outside and find a comfortable place to sit.

Notice the earth—maybe touch the ground and feel it. What does the earth have to teach you about awareness reflected in yourself?

- The earth can represent the concept of solidity or steadfastness. It is the ground from which everything arises, emerges, falls away, and arises again. It supports all phenomena, regardless of form, without preference. The earth has no judgment about which plants will grow, or where or how. The earth has no judgment about the height or location of a mountain or the depths of a canyon.
- The earth is also allowing. Notice the various plants that emerge from the earth, consider again the ascent of mountains, the descent of canyons. The earth symbolizes that quality of awareness that can teach us to allow for the continuous arising and falling away—birth, growth, decay—of all thoughts, emotions, beliefs, and identity. The earth simply allows for all things to arise, to be supported and nourished, and receives them back to rise again as something new.
- The earth teaches us this quality of awareness that allows, provides space for, and nourishes all things. It holds the space for cracks, crevices, movement, and mountains without judgment. It can teach us how to be with any stimulus without preference, and to continue to support and assimilate what arises and what falls away.

Bring the intention of understanding this quality of awareness that is the earth into your experience of your body. Scan your body. Can you allow, nourish, and support all arising sensations? Can you find that quality of awareness that allows all sensations to arise without judgment or preference? That allows sensations to be nourished and supported? The substrate from which one sensation diminishing becomes another arising? The substrate from which we can give space to all sensation, no matter how difficult, joyful, wonderful, or harsh?

Bring to the mind an intention to understand this quality of awareness that is the earth. Notice thoughts, emotions, and beliefs that arise. What happens if you connect to the quality of awareness that is steadfastly accepting, allowing, supportive, and nourishing, that can both give and receive back all of what is offered and seen?

Practice 5.3 Body, Mind, and Environment Reflecting Awareness—Water

Repeat the exercise in Practice 5.2 with water. Find a body of water to contemplate. Notice the qualities that water has to teach you about awareness reflected within yourself.

- Water is fluid and dynamic. When water meets obstacles, it simply moves around or through them. Over time, water can even wear down obstacles such as rocks or earth—it embodies qualities of patience and abiding.
- Water also maintains its essence. No matter what rides on its surface or resides within it, the water itself is unchanged.
- How is this reflected in the experience of your body? How is your body fluid, patient, and abiding? What happens when you connect to this aspect of your body that is dynamic yet retains its essence?
- How is this reflected in the experience of your mind? How are your thoughts, emotions, and beliefs fluid, patient, and abiding? What happens when you connect to this aspect of your mind that is dynamic and yet retains its essence?

Practice 5.4 Body, Mind, and Environment Reflecting Awareness—Fire

Repeat the exercise in Practice 5.2 with the element of fire. Find a candle to contemplate. What qualities inherent to fire can teach you about awareness reflected within yourself?

- Fire illuminates, but it also promotes growth for beings and plants. Fire also transforms one thing into another; it is a catalyst. Transformation happens through the heat of fire, just as anything held in the light of awareness changes.
- How do you experience these qualities of illumination, growth, and transformation in your body? What happens when you connect physically to these qualities?
- How are these qualities reflected in the experience of your mind? What happens when you connect to these qualities within your thoughts, emotions, and beliefs?

Practice 5.5 Body, Mind, and Environment Reflecting Awareness—Wind

Repeat the exercise in Practice 5.2 with wind. Find a place to sit and feel the air on your body. What qualities inherent to the wind can teach you about awareness reflected in yourself?

- Wind moves dynamically and can carry along objects.
- How are these qualities of movement and transport reflected in your body? What happens when you connect physically to these qualities?
- How are these qualities reflected in the experience of your mind? What happens when you connect to dynamism and the movement of thoughts, emotions, and beliefs?

Practice 5.6 Body, Mind, and Environment Reflecting Awareness—Space

Repeat the exercise in Practice 5.2 with space. Notice the space around and between things. What qualities inherent to space can teach you about awareness reflected in yourself?

- Space extends into everything; it is within and between things. The space between objects gives them their form and shape.
- How is this quality of space reflected in your body, and what happens as you connect to the space within it?
- How is this quality of space reflected in your mind, and what happens as you connect to the space between thoughts, emotions, and beliefs?

Conclusion

A New Look at the Burning of the Khandava Forest

With this information about prana, the subtle body, and tantra we can explore the symbolism of the story from the beginning of the chapter. Its metaphors can help us move beyond conceptualization or intellectualization of the teachings to entextualization—the teachings become an embodied experience.

In this story, Agni symbolizes prana, our vital energy. He has been poisoned, diminishing his strength and luster. In much the same way, our own vitality can become depleted, or it can be supported and enlivened. Our level of vitality can be affected by such varied sources as the types of food we eat; the quality of our sleep; musculoskeletal and postural imbalances; physical activity; the quality of thoughts, emotions, and beliefs; and the environment we inhabit, including the people and situations we encounter.

When we work with clients, we can see this diminished vitality in their experience of pain, chronic illness, negative states of mind, interpersonal relationships, or external situations. Each of these factors can become a stressor resulting in diminished physical and/or mental health.

Agni is poisoned by a greedy king who wants to perform an elaborate ceremony for his own benefit, without considering the repercussions of his actions. The greedy king represents the mind (thoughts and emotions—manas and ahamkara) blinded to truth through misperception or ignorance. In this story, the individual's vitality (agni) is being diminished as their actions are ruled by the misperceptions of the mind—heedless of the impact of these actions on themselves or on others. This disregard for the effects of one's actions is the very opposite of the yogic emphasis on harmony and dharma.

The term *adharma* signifies actions that go against the harmony among oneself, others, and one's environment. Agni's story teaches that when we oppose dharma, we lose vitality, strength, and connection to our essential nature. Agni's lost vitality is the lost well-being resulting from adharmic action.

When Agni is sick, he seeks Brahman's guidance about what he needs to heal and restore his nature. Brahman represents awareness, and thus the story emphasizes that it is through connecting to one's inner essence as awareness that wisdom and insight emerge. Through self-reflection and self-inquiry, we can discover both the sources of depletion and what we need to recover and flourish. This capacity for self-discovery and ultimately self-empowerment in the healing process is a foundational concept of yoga therapy.

Brahman tells Agni that a very particular forest, along with its inhabitants, holds the key to the restoration of his health. The Khandava Forest and its unfamiliar creatures symbolize an unexplored place within the subtle body—a granthi or chakra, representing unexamined tensions and disconnections for the yogi to contemplate. The yogi must resolve these relationships to body sensations, thoughts, emotions, or beliefs to connect to the fullness of who they are, to their optimal vitality.

This kind of disconnection, even from one's essential nature, often occurs in various therapeutic populations including those with pain, trauma, or chronic illness. The body can become a source of betrayal, grief, sadness, or anger. The person may choose to shut off from emotional or cognitive experiences—for example, grief or even great joy—if they seem threatening or overwhelming. An antagonistic relationship can develop, resulting in shutting off from, disregarding, or disdaining one's own body and mind.

Any of these unresolved physical or psychoemotional experiences becomes a "forest" in the subtle body, and the various physical, psychological, and behavioral phenomena requiring exploration are the creatures within. Just as the inhabitants of the Khandava Forest are described as the "enemies of the gods," unexamined tensions and relationships oppose the person's connection to their essential nature as awareness. The subtle body thus becomes a map for the exploration of our inner terrain; through meditative yoga practices, we can use this map to find places of disconnection from our true nature.

Agni, fire, illuminates the forests. Fire is also an element of transformation—heat can alter the very structure of material from one form into another. Awareness has a similar capacity for transforming our habitual way of relating to physical, mental, and environmental phenomena. Shifts occur when we become the compassionate observer of these stimuli, able to hold them inside a container of equanimity, contentment, and the steadfast joy of awareness. Rather than misidentifying with these stimuli, we can learn our habitual patterns of reaction to discern right action and restore vitality and well-being.

When we hold what lies within the forests—granthis or chakras—inside the container of awareness, a kind of alchemy occurs. Experiences like anger, sadness, or grief can be observed alongside the qualities that emerge from awareness. This capacity creates new patterns of relationship with such experiences. The knots disentangle as the light of awareness pierces through the granthis' obscuration. We are able to accept all aspects of our being, connecting deeply to awareness amidst fluctuating phenomena.

In this story, each time Agni tries to consume the Khandava Forest, Indra thwarts him. Indra, the king of the gods, represents the aspect of ourselves that seeks to protect ego structures, such as core beliefs and habitual patterns, to maintain a sense of individuality. The king of the serpents, one of the "friends" Indra wants to protect, represents the core beliefs that form the foundation of our identities.

These structures of belief and identity create a sense of safety and familiarity for the mind and ego. The concept of dissolving this sense of identity, changing core beliefs and habits, endangers the status quo. Indra therefore extinguishes any threat to identity—his rains symbolize the obstacles that arise as we dive into a process of discovery. These obstacles might include overpowering physical sensations, thoughts, emotions, or beliefs.

Each time the individual begins to explore the subtle body and uncover these core beliefs, the mind and ego work to protect a sense of safety, individuality, and separateness. Agni tries to illuminate what is within, but insight is obscured and vitality diminished. Indra works to protect these habitual patterns of relationship to body, mind, and environment—areas of experience that the person has not examined or may not be ready to explore.

Brahman advises Agni to seek out both Arjuna and Krishna to help consume the Khandava Forest. The importance of the relationship between Arjuna and Krishna is a recurrent theme in the Mahabharata and in the Bhagavad Gita contained therein. As previously noted, Arjuna represents the archetypical warrior and the discipline of the yoga practices. Krishna represents our true nature as awareness. Both must work together to restore Agni's health; Arjuna and Krishna complement each other just as discipline and the realization of awareness work together to restore vitality and well-being.

Discipline (Arjuna) enables the structure and clarity needed to be with the stimuli of the body, mind, and environment without becoming overwhelmed or overidentified with them. At the same time, the recognition of all phenomena as awareness (Krishna) empowers us to notice everything that arises with equanimity, contentment, and steadfast joy. This balance of discipline and welcoming of stimuli provides the insight to discern right action in synchrony with our surroundings; dharma is realized through alignment of discipline with awareness. The importance of this relationship is highlighted again at the end of the story when Krishna asks for no reward other than eternal friendship with Arjuna.

The yoga practices themselves serve as the disciplined practice through which physical, mental, and environmental phenomena can be understood as awareness. Arjuna and Krishna tirelessly circle the forest's perimeter. The discipline of the practices held in the light of awareness allows the yogi to avoid being misdirected by anything that emerges from the forest. As the yogi focuses, no matter what thought, sensation, emotion, or belief emerges he is able to maintain the integrity of the practice in the light of compassionate observation, nonjudgmental attention, and equanimity. Regardless of how much Indra's rains or the mind's resistance try to distract the yogi, he continues to illuminate the forests inside. Vitality and prana are restored to those dark, obstructed places, and the yogi is able to continue the practice as the clarity of deep awareness strengthens.

Ultimately, Agni consumes the forest; prana pierces through the obscurations and obstacles of the granthis or chakras. We become more resilient, well-integrated in our capacity to abide with the wide spectrum of sensation, emotion, thought, and belief. Indra, as father to Arjuna, is proud of this feat. The mind that feared the prana and realization of awareness, once overthrown, finds qualities of contentment, equanimity, and steadfast joy within that very awareness.

> **Practice 5.7 Meditation on the Khandava Forest**
>
> Lie or sit in a comfortable position. Allow the body to settle and the mind to be free to wander.
>
> Find an image or word that can represent the discipline to return to a sense of comfort, peace, equanimity, or calm. As you move through this meditation, when sensation begins to overwhelm the mind or body, come back to this image or word—to this facet of awareness that is peace or comfort. This is the linking of Arjuna and Krishna—discipline and awareness.
>
> Begin to explore inner sensation. Notice a place that may be unknown, dark, obscured—a forest. Notice how your sense of vitality may be diminished here, your connection to awareness obscured. Notice the quality of physical sensation—color, texture, vibration. Notice the kinds of thoughts, emotions, and beliefs that arise as you explore this area. Notice how the mind might create, from these sensations, an experience that takes you away from the present moment.
>
> Visualize this space inside as a forest. Find a breath technique, movement, or position that draws your attention here. Visualize Arjuna and Krishna circumambulating this forest, building a tent of arrows to shield it from the mind. Bring in the image or word from the beginning to become this tent of arrows. Notice the nonconceptual part of the experience—colors, texture, vibration, sound—all of these experiences underneath the mind trying to create concept or story. Every time a thought, belief, or emotion arises—like a creature trying to escape—return to bodily sensation, color, texture, image, vibration, sound. Bring alongside any distraction the image of peace, comfort, or equanimity.
>
> Illuminate this space by maintaining focus, with a posture or breathing technique that draws attention here (Arjuna, the discipline of the practice), and by welcoming all sensation as awareness (Krishna). Allow this process until a natural softening and resolution of experience occur. Notice whether you sense calm and equanimity as the mind lets go into spaciousness and allowing.

Notes

1. Dharma, K. (1999). *Mahabharata: The greatest spiritual epic of all time.* Badger, CA: Torchlight Publishing; Ganguli, K. M. (2001). *The Mahabharata* (Vol. 3). New Delhi: Munshiram Manoharlal; Smith, J. D. (Ed.). (2009). *The Mahabharata.* London: Penguin Classics.
2. Mallinson, J., & Singleton, M. (2017). *Roots of yoga.* London: Penguin.
3. *The Upanishads* (Vol. 2), translated by Eknath Easwaran, founder of the Blue Mountain Center of Meditation, copyright 1987, 2007; reprinted by permission of Nilgiri Press, P. O. Box 256, Tomales, CA 94971, www.bmcm.org.
4. Easwaran, *The Upanishads.*
5. Easwaran, *The Upanishads.*
6. Finlayson, D. (2018, December 20). A yoga therapy perspective on the human system: The panchamaya model [blog]. Retrieved from https://yogatherapy.health/2018/12/20/a-yoga-therapy-perspective-on-the-human-system-the-panchamaya-model/
7. Wallis, C. D. (2012). *Tantra illuminated: The philosophy, history, and practice of a timeless tradition*, p. 133. The Woodlands, TX: Anusara Press.
8. Finlayson, A yoga therapy perspective on the human system.
9. Wallis, *Tantra illuminated.*
10. Mallinson & Singleton, *Roots of yoga.*
11. Mallinson & Singleton, *Roots of yoga.*
12. Mallinson & Singleton, *Roots of yoga.*
13. Mallinson & Singleton, *Roots of yoga.*
14. Wallis, *Tantra illuminated.*
15. Mallinson & Singleton, *Roots of yoga*; Flood, G. (2005). *The tantric body: The secret tradition of Hindu religion.* London: I.B. Tauris.
16. Mallinson & Singleton, *Roots of yoga*; Flood, *The tantric body*; Wallis, *Tantra illuminated.*
17. Flood, *The tantric body*; Wallis, *Tantra illuminated.*
18. Wallis, *Tantra illuminated*, p. 26.
19. Miller, R. (2015). *Level I training manual*, p. 3, Integrative Restoration Institute. San Rafael, CA: iRest Institute.
20. Personal correspondence, Richard Miller, April 1, 2019
21. Wallis, *Tantra illuminated.*
22. Flood, *The tantric body.*
23. Flood, *The tantric body.*
24. Mallinson & Singleton, *Roots of yoga.*
25. Flood, *The tantric body.*
26. Flood, *The tantric body*; Mallinson & Singleton, *Roots of yoga.*
27. Flood, *The tantric body.*
28. Flood, *The tantric body*, p. 4.
29. Flood, *The tantric body.*

PART II

Exploring Theoretical and Explanatory Frameworks for Yoga Therapy as an Integrative Healthcare Practice

Explanatory Model for Yoga Therapy to Promote Health and Well-Being   6

The biomedical model focuses on treating diseases that can be explained by a particular pathogen or physiological mechanism. Although this model is incredibly valuable, it has its limitations. Throughout history, models that considered different factors have been used to understand states of health and disease.

The yogic kosha model described in Chapter 5 offers one perspective for exploring the layers of an individual's experience including the physical, energetic, psychoemotional, and spiritual. This model is similar to one used in integrative and complementary healthcare, the biopsychosocial-spiritual (BPSS) model. The BPSS model helps us explore the complexity of health and well-being as a dynamic relationship within multidimensional human experience. With growing research showing the significance of social and spiritual contributors to health, the BPSS model has gained recognition and acceptance in healthcare contexts.

Both ancient paradigms, such as the koshas, and contemporary ones, such as the BPSS model, help us to understand that the state of our health results from the ever-changing expression of multiple domains of experience. Every person we meet represents a unique puzzle of each domain's expression and patterns of interaction. As we help clients explore their own puzzles, we can help them to understand the roots of their suffering or pain and facilitate its alleviation, empowering them to access their own capacity for well-being.

Rather than reducing the human experience to one or two components, the BPSS and kosha models enable investigation of each layer's contribution to states of health and well-being or to illness, pain, and suffering. Considering these spheres independently and in relationship offers a way to comprehensively understand an individual's experience in health and well-being.

This chapter's movement between ancient yogic and contemporary integrative health models is meant to provide a translational language. Such shared languages enhance the accessibility of traditional philosophies to current healthcare contexts, including research, and work with individual clients. To be clear, we do not intend to reduce one model to the other, but rather to draw helpful convergences and parallels for accessibility and use in different contexts.

Domains of Health and Well-Being and the Koshas

Physical Domain and Annamaya/Pranamaya Kosha

The physical domain of health is composed of the gross materiality of annamaya (the structures of the systems of the body, including bones, muscles, blood vessels, and organs) as well as pranamaya (the physiological functioning of these systems, providing energy and vitality as described in Chapter 5).

Psychological Domain and Manomaya/Vijnanamaya Kosha

The psychological domain of health includes various components of mental/emotional experience such as cognition, intellect, emotion, and mood. Experience in this domain is affected by our capacity to understand concepts and process information, ability to synthesize and develop ideas, proficiency in recognizing and identifying feelings and emotions, and ability to manage mood and emotion.

This domain of health is reflected in the yogic kosha of manomaya, including manas and ahamkara. It also includes aspects of vijnanamaya in the capacity for discernment and around beliefs.

Social Domain and Vijnanamaya/Anandamaya Kosha

The social domain of health includes our capacity to engage in healthy relationships, form connections, trust, and interact with others in meaningful ways.

Although the koshas may not have a direct parallel to this domain of health, the attributes of vijnanamaya and anandamaya influence the development of quality social relationships. From vijnanamaya kosha, insight into our habitual patterns may help us discover how thoughts, emotions, and behavior facilitate or hinder healthy social connection. Pitfalls such as lack of trust or inability to connect with others can be explored through discernment and inquiry. In addition, working with the yamas and niyamas (ethical principles) to develop attributes such as patience, acceptance, contentment, and nonharming can promote healthier relationships.

Anandamaya kosha also influences the development of healthy social connections. The realization of one's essential nature as awareness changes the way we interact with others, fostering relationships from a foundation of contentment, equanimity, and steadfast joy. The realization of shared awareness within all beings supports the recognition of our inherent interconnection. This understanding can assist the emergence of prosocial behaviors like compassion and empathy.

Spiritual Domain and Anandamaya Kosha

Common themes found in spiritual traditions include meaning and purpose; a sense of connectedness that could involve the present moment, internal resourcing, other people, nature, and the transcendent/existential; emphasis on cultivating positive psychological and behavioral attributes (e.g., hope, optimism, compassion); positive reappraisal of life situations including meaning-making; and social support.[1]

Yoga's spiritual tradition shares many of these themes as foundational to its philosophy. Meaning and purpose are reflected in ideas of dharma. A sense of connectedness is taught through the realization of one's essential nature as awareness. This recognition emphasizes the shared awareness that extends to others and to transcendent/existential connectedness. A focus on the yamas and niyamas mirrors the importance of cultivating positive traits like contentment, patience, and nonharming. Anandamaya kosha provides a window through which meaning, connectedness, and positive psychological/behavioral traits emerge.

Shifting the Paradigm to Interconnection, From Static to Dynamic

The BPSS components of health are not meant to be understood as silos of distinct experiences, but rather as interrelated spheres that influence one another in creating an individual's present-moment experience and state of health or well-being. These relationships are dynamically intertwined, as each domain constantly fluctuates and affects the others. Health and well-being can therefore be described more accurately as a process, a fluid interplay. The physical, psychological, social, and spiritual aspects of our experience are engaged in a dynamic dance, influencing one another in the experience of health and well-being or pain, illness, and suffering.

Recognizing that these domains are dynamically interrelated helps us to work with health and well-being in a way that honors the complex layers of experience. The domains' constantly shifting movement reflects who we are, and insight into pain, meaning, and experience depends on our understanding of what is happening within these dimensions of health and well-being. Yoga therapy has a unique, important role in addressing the domains of health concurrently, within a cohesive and comprehensive philosophical methodology.

A Closer Look at the Social and Spiritual Domains of Health

Despite their intangibility, the social and spiritual domains significantly influence health and well-being. These domains are especially relevant to the framework of yoga therapy as a distinct practice. Before we dive into more psychophysiological theoretical frameworks in Chapter 7, we will consider the research behind the significance of the social and spiritual domains.

The Social Domain's Influence on Health and Well-Being

The social domain of health has to do with a sense of connection to others and emphasizes the quality of relationships, which in turn involve the development of prosocial attributes and virtues essential for healthy interactions. Importantly, it is the *quality*, not the *quantity*, of relationships and social connections that significantly influences health and well-being.

In research, this distinction is termed *objective* versus *perceived* social isolation to reflect quantity versus quality, respectively. Objective isolation depends on factors such as number, proximity, or frequency of social interactions and relationships. Perceived social isolation depends on feelings such as loneliness or isolation and on the presence of meaningful relationships. Perceived, rather than objective, social isolation has significant adverse health effects. Perceived social isolation is a risk factor for broad-based mortality and morbidity (e.g., high blood pressure, Alzheimer's disease); increases depressive symptoms; negatively affects inflammatory and immune processes; decreases physical function and increases disability in chronic conditions; and affects the experience of pain (interference, levels of distress, severity, and adjustment).[2] The considerable and widespread mental and physical health effects of perceived isolation demonstrate the need to address this domain in various patient populations for optimal well-being.

The Spiritual Domain's Influence on Health and Well-Being

The spiritual domain of health is assessed through measures that evaluate themes including those mentioned above: meaning and purpose, sense of connectedness, positive psychological and behavioral attributes, and social support.

Growing evidence links health in the spiritual domain to positive health outcomes, including improved experience of pain (severity, tolerance, sensitivity), coping and adjustment to chronic pain and illness, quality of life, symptoms of anxiety and depression, systemic physical health (cardiovascular, endocrine, immunity), mortality and morbidity, and social support. In particular, meaning and purpose have been linked to significant positive health outcomes such as decreased all-cause mortality, improved inflammatory and immune processes, enhanced well-being and functioning in chronic pain conditions, lower pain intensity and pain interference with activities, and lower pain-medication use.[3] The spiritual domain's significant consequences for physical, mental, and social health demonstrate the importance of identifying interventions that support spiritual well-being.

Eudaimonic Well-Being and the Spiritual Domain of Health

Spiritual and eudaimonic well-being share characteristics of meaning and purpose, virtues, and quality social relationships (see Figure 6.1). Eudaimonic and spiritual well-being also have unique features that both differentiate them and demonstrate their influence on each other. Eudaimonic well-being includes the distinct traits of self-realization, self-actualization, personal expressiveness, integrity, and authenticity. Spiritual well-being includes a specific focus on personal and/or transcendent existential connection.

118 Theoretical and Explanatory Frameworks

SPIRITUAL TEACHINGS | **EUDAIMONIC WELL-BEING**

- Meaning/purpose
- Virtues
- Interpersonal connection: social relationships

- Personal connection
- Transcendental/ existential connection

- Self-realization/ self-actualization
- Authenticity, integrity, personal expressiveness

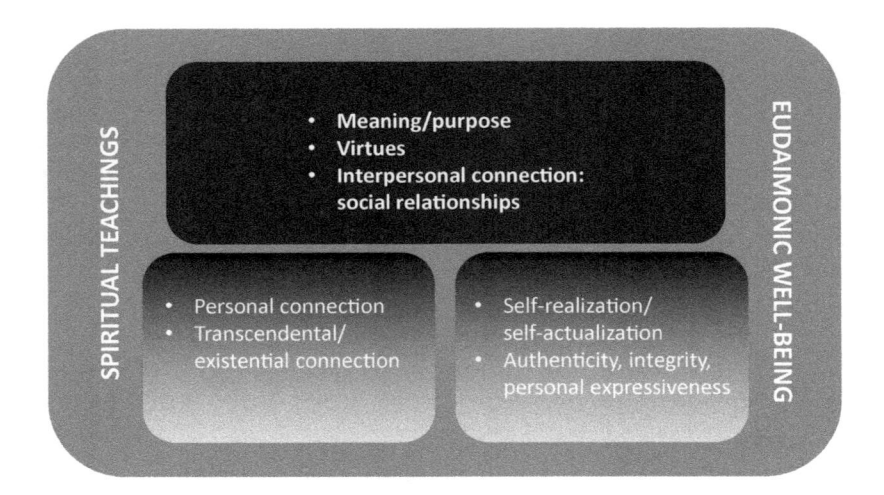

Figure 6.1 Similarities and Parallels in Spiritual and Eudaimonic Teachings.

Note: Directly aligned themes (top), and unique but mutually influential and supportive themes of spiritual teachings (left) and eudaimonic well-being (right).

The personal connectedness of spiritual teachings may foster the self-actualization, personal expressiveness, and authenticity of eudaimonic well-being and vice versa. Yoga includes teachings through which we realize our essential nature as awareness and connect to this deeper understanding of who we are beneath the fluctuations of the body, mind, and habitual tendencies. As we come to understand and connect to this deeper aspect of ourselves (from a spiritual lens), we can live and express ourselves more authentically (from a eudaimonic lens).

The transcendent or existential connection found in spiritual teachings can support eudaimonic ideas of meaning, purpose, self-realization, and self-actualization. Existential or transcendental connection can encourage constructive and positive reflection on life events. A positive reappraisal of circumstances fosters meaning-making, and self-reflection facilitates personal growth and development. The process of self-discovery encourages eudaimonic attributes such as personal expression, authenticity, and ultimately self-actualization as we learn to connect to life in a way that helps us to flourish and realize our potential.

Portals to Entry

Working with any aspect of eudaimonic or spiritual well-being can influence or encourage the development of the others (Figure 6.2). These relationships

Explanatory Model for Yoga Therapy 119

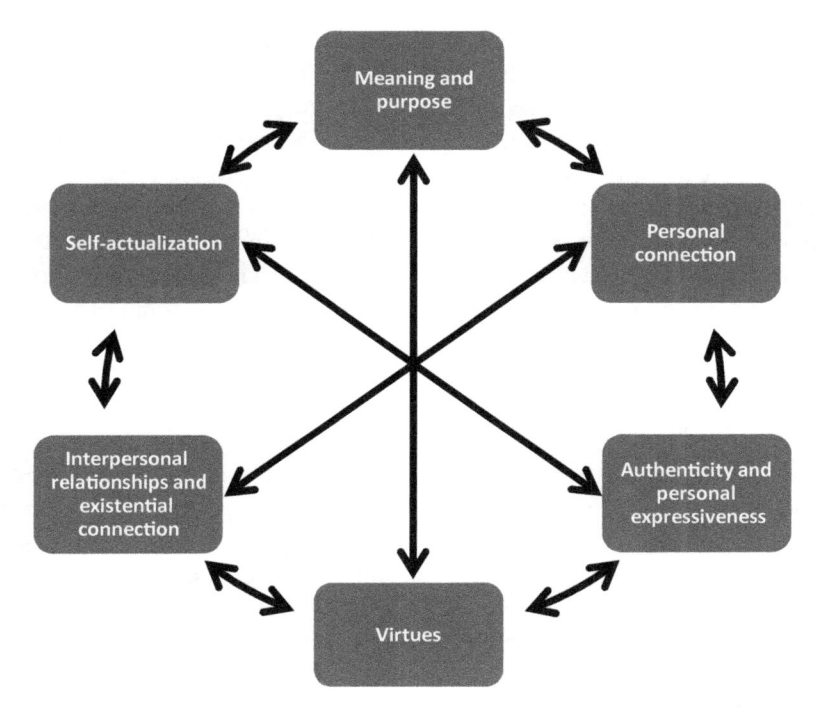

Figure 6.2 Relationships Between Eudaimonic and Spiritual Components of Well-Being.

Note: Any component can be the starting point, and each mutually supports the development of the others, synchronously or subsequently, for improved well-being.

are nonlinear: Any component of well-being can serve as the starting point and affect the others in a multitude of ways along synchronous or consecutive pathways; we will explore several possible entry points here.

Meaning and Purpose

Meaning and purpose represent an important shared theme with significant influence on the other components of spirituality and eudaimonia, as well as on health outcomes (including pain, mortality, inflammation and immune processes, and pain-medication use, as stated above). With its considerable effect on physical, mental, social, and spiritual domains, meaning is an essential foundation for a holistic perspective on health and well-being. As such, it is important to find accessible ways to bring the topic into client care. Yoga therapy is ideal for this work, as meaning and purpose are central to its explanatory framework and it provides a methodology for inquiring into them.

Contemplating meaning and purpose in life situations can help us find a greater intrapersonal connection to our truth, values, and needs. We are then able to authentically express ourselves with integrity to these values. The virtues, as described below, are inherent to understanding values and needs and to assist with the reflection necessary to determine right action. Authentic action results in better quality interpersonal relationships and in connection to life or something greater. This positive cycle facilitates meaning-making amidst adversity to help promote a more constructive view of ourselves and our lives. The whole process helps us to fulfill our highest potential and to become self-actualized, enhancing a sense of meaning and purpose and thus propagating the cycle.

Virtues and Ethical Inquiry

The philosophy of eudaimonia includes an emphasis on the virtue ethics as guideposts along the route toward its fulfillment. According to the theory of the virtue ethics, reflection on and practice of these moral characteristics engenders right action, leading to a well-lived, purposeful life—a life of eudaimonia.

Spiritual teachings also often include a process for reflection on and promotion of certain qualities or virtues such as love, awe, joy, forgiveness, hope, gratitude, honesty, patience, and compassion.[4] These virtues are taught as ways to facilitate more meaningful and positive relationships and to cultivate more constructive intrapersonal, interpersonal, and existential connections.

Like meaning and purpose, the virtues are important to both spirituality and eudaimonic well-being and affect the other components of these teachings (see Figure 6.2). Through the lens of spiritual teachings, work with these qualities helps to cultivate intrapersonal connection as we discover a healthier perspective on our self-concept, body-mind state, and experience of wellness (or unwellness). From a sense of interpersonal connection, we find different ways of interacting with others to include greater patience, tolerance, and so on, in turn facilitating ever more meaningful relationships. Transcendental connection also arises from these qualities, as they help us to reappraise situations, such as chronic pain or other health conditions, to adopt more constructive and adaptive perspectives on life situations. This reflection can also foster greater meaning and purpose in the face of challenging circumstances.

Through the lens of eudaimonic well-being, the virtues can facilitate self-actualization. Reflection on the virtue ethics helps us to uncover the most authentic expression of ourselves, live to our highest potential, and discover meaning and purpose. Ultimately, these virtues include an inquiry into qualities that promote better connections to ourselves, others, and life circumstances.

As discussed in Chapter 2, central to yoga philosophy and practice are the yamas and niyamas. These ethical principles are the doorways to dharma, the guideposts to right action in difficult life situations. The yamas and niyamas, like dharma, are fundamental to the explanatory framework of yoga therapy. Yoga teaches principles such as nonharming, contentment, and truthfulness for reflection and as characteristics that naturally emerge from the realization of one's essential nature as awareness.

Self-Actualization

The concept of self-actualization could be considered the epitome of the well-lived life described by eudaimonia, as the latter can include the development of an individual's highest potential. Chapter 3 examines Viktor Frankl's teaching that life presents the opportunity for finding meaning in our responses to each moment. According to yogic philosophy, too, our responses to life contain the seeds of growth, development of our strengths, understanding of our limitations, and ultimately self-actualization.

We are shaped by our reactions to life, which enable us to embody our intentions. For example, if a person wants to develop kindness or compassion, she might examine a trying situation in her life. Reflecting on kindness or compassion, she could discern the kinds of actions needed to meet the difficult circumstance in a way that actualizes that particular virtue.

A person with a chronic condition may habitually respond to flareups by berating himself, feeling betrayed by his body or the world, or feeling angry at those around him when they do not understand the condition. This individual could instead contemplate what meeting the flareup with kindness or compassion entails, reflecting on what would be required to be fully present to the experience while being compassionate to himself, others, and in relationship to life circumstances. This might mean making time for more rest, not taking on as much work, or conserving energy resources by carefully choosing with whom and with what to become involved.

Contemplating a virtue like kindness in a situation such as a flareup, illness, or pain can help to create meaning from difficulty. This provides an opportunity for personal growth as we learn to consider adversity through a lens of transformation. The process of reappraisal empowers us to see our gifts and our strengths as we learn to relate to perceived limitations differently. We are able to flourish and realize the highest expression of ourselves even in unpleasant situations. In this way, life situations like an illness help us move from theoretical concepts to practical application. Ultimately, the process of reflecting on what is arising in the present moment, deciding how to meet it from the perspective of the virtues, then acting from that perspective empowers us to find meaning, develop to our highest potential, and find purpose within an illness situation. This reflective decision-making and action are integral to yoga's philosophical and ethical foundations.

Self-actualization can be related to the spiritual teaching of connecting to one's highest self—a sense of internal wisdom, resource, or guidance. Reflecting on and developing our gifts naturally deepens self-understanding. Yogic teachings and practices can facilitate this process of discovery of our essential nature as we learn to disentangle from the fluctuations of the psychophysiological and worldly constituents of prakriti and connect to awareness within. This realization of ourselves as awareness can be understood as the pinnacle of self-actualization.

Clinical Relevance

The overlap between these definitions of spirituality and eudaimonic well-being has provided a fruitful contribution to my work with clients, helping me to develop my own language to open the door for these important discussions. I attribute many clients' most powerful "healing moments," through which transformative realizations occurred, to these conversations.

Clients are supported through dialogue and inquiry to express these concepts in relation to their own values for their unique healing journeys. Opportunities for personal expression of spirituality arise from these conversations, without the client feeling pushed into or triggered by either religious or spiritual topics. This is the epitome of client-centered care—offering people the opportunity to reflect upon and determine how these concepts show up for them, defining the ideas in a way that supports their healing and well-being.

Understanding the language and research behind spiritual and eudaimonic well-being is also valuable in presenting yoga therapy ideas to allopathic medical professionals. This translational language clarifies the importance of these concepts for clinical care while increasing their accessibility to healthcare providers.

The Health Effects of Eudaimonic Well-Being

Significant research supports the important positive effects of eudaimonic well-being on physical and mental health.

- Eudaimonic well-being has demonstrated a positive effect on inflammatory and immune processes, including compensating for the negative effect of perceived social isolation on these factors seen in cancer, neurodegenerative, and cardiovascular disease states.[5] Furthermore, the effect of eudaimonic well-being on the gene profile responsible for these results has been found to be independent of other demographic and health variables.[6] This genomic expression is also sensitive to hedonic versus eudaimonic well-being. Although both types of well-being show similar affective outcomes, eudaimonic well-being downregulates this gene profile while hedonic happiness upregulates it.[7]
- Eudaimonic well-being is associated with decreased levels of salivary cortisol, proinflammatory cytokines, and cardiovascular disease risk, but hedonic happiness has minimal effect on these biomarkers.[8]
- In people who report greater eudaimonic well-being, negative stimuli prompt less amygdala activation and more engagement of higher cortical structures. This demonstrates a potential capacity for greater discernment to transform habitual reactions to more constructive behaviors in the presence of greater eudaimonic well-being. In addition, sustained activation of reward circuitry has been found in response to positive stimuli in those who report eudaimonic well-being.[9]
- The absence of eudaimonic well-being increases the probability of all-cause mortality independent of factors such as age, gender, race, physical inactivity, and conditions such as cardiovascular disease, cancer, or stroke.[10]
- In chronic pain conditions, eudaimonic well-being is related to lower levels of fatigue, disability, pain intensity, and pain-medication use and to improved well-being, patient functioning, adjustment to chronic pain, depression symptoms, and life satisfaction.[11]

This research illuminates the need to find interventions to address this significant contributor to health. As discussed above, themes of eudaimonic well-being are both shared with and complementary to those of spirituality and can help these ideas become more accessible in clinical care. Yoga shares these themes as foundational to its explanatory framework and may therefore provide a methodology through which they can be integrated into interventions for various client populations. Understanding eudaimonic and spiritual well-being as central to yoga's methodology may help clients, healthcare professionals, and researchers understand the unique purview of yoga therapy in healthcare settings.

> **Practice 6.1 Journaling on Eudaimonic or Spiritual Well-Being**
>
> Choose one of these concepts:
>
> - meaning and purpose;
> - virtues (e.g., contentment, nonharming);
> - interpersonal connection/social relationships;
> - self-realization or self-actualization;
> - authenticity, integrity, personal expressiveness/personal connection; or
> - existential or transcendental connection.
>
> Reflect on what the concept means to you. These ideas may show up differently throughout our lives as our sense of ourselves changes and different circumstances arise. How has this concept shown up in your life? How would you like it to show up in your life?
>
> How do you see the concept you chose affecting the other concepts, both directly and indirectly?
>
> How might you embody the concepts in your daily life?
>
> Try to spend a day focusing on your chosen concept, and notice how it affects the others. Notice also how it affects your relationship to your body, mind, and life situations.

Yoga Therapy as an Integrative Healthcare Practice

Yoga therapy combines modern evidence-based and traditional practices to offer a comprehensive methodology that addresses individuals' BPSS concerns. Understanding yogic practices within this integrated, systematic framework is essential to appreciate yoga therapy's potential effectiveness as a distinct complementary and integrative healthcare profession.

When yoga therapy practices are broken apart, delivered in isolation from one another, reduced to constituent parts, or not given to further an intention of alleviating suffering and promoting eudaimonic well-being, we can expect that their effectiveness may be limited. This reductionist approach occurs when asana is simply given for muscular or joint imbalances, breath techniques only for autonomic nervous system regulation, or meditations only for mood and emotional regulation. The practice becomes akin to a form of physical rehabilitation with exercise prescription, stress-management, or mindfulness programs provided within a biomedical framework. Although these may all be beneficial practices, they differ from yoga or yoga therapy. To define yoga therapy as any one of these components, or solely within a biomedical framework, diminishes its intent and potential. This limited application can also create misunderstandings that leave medical professionals, researchers, and the public unable to discern the distinctiveness of and need for yoga therapy in client care.

Yoga Therapy's Explanatory Framework

Foundational to yoga therapy is the perspective that the individual's relationship to their body, mind, and environment is the cause of suffering in pain, illness, or disability.[12] Reconnection to our nature as awareness is essential to the alleviation of suffering. From this realization, we can experience an underlying contentment, equanimity, and eudaimonic well-being even amidst pain, illness, or disability. We discover inner and outer harmony (dharma) as we are supported to reflect on the actions—including ways of thinking and interacting with oneself, others, and life—that promote this alignment. Ethical inquiry and discriminative wisdom are essential practices for cultivating the insight to transform habitual relationships with the body, mind, and environment to more constructive ones that foster eudaimonic well-being (see Figure 6.3).

Components of spiritual and eudaimonic well-being, such as meaning and purpose, virtues, and personal and existential/transcendental connectedness are at the core of yoga therapy's model. Other components of spiritual and eudaimonic well-being, including quality social relationships, authenticity, and self-actualization, develop from the philosophical and theoretical teachings of yoga. As we gain insight into our personal values to understand our most authentic selves, we learn to act with integrity to these values and to interact with others in healthier, more meaningful ways to fulfill our potential and flourish.

Asana, meditation, and other yoga therapy practices can be provided in the context of this framework, oriented to facilitate spiritual and eudaimonic well-being. Using movement as an example, asana offers a way to both explore habits of the mind and body as well as to embody new experiences. An individual may come to yoga therapy with the intention of creating greater ease or calm in the body and mind. Movement may prompt discomfort or agitation, so the yoga therapist can aid in identifying movement that instead expresses calm or ease. The person learns to identify this spectrum from calm to agitation as well as the capacity to move between the two

126 Theoretical and Explanatory Frameworks

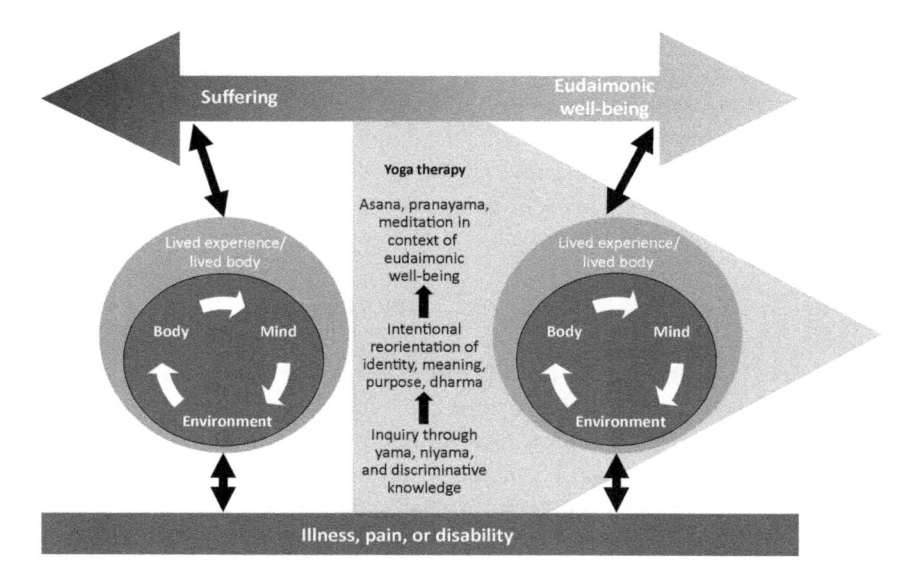

Figure 6.3 Yoga Therapy's Explanatory Framework.

Note: The experience of pain, illness, or disability can shift our relationship to body, mind, and environment toward suffering. Likewise, suffering can create a relationship with the body, mind, and environment that perpetuates illness, pain, or disability. Yoga therapy cultivates discriminative wisdom, ethical inquiry, and right action in alignment with meaning and purpose to shift these relationships toward eudaimonic well-being, regardless of circumstance.

Source: Adapted from Sullivan, M. B., Moonaz, S., Weber, K., Taylor, J. N., & Schmalzl, L. (2018). Toward an explanatory framework for yoga therapy informed by philosophical and ethical perspectives. *Alternative Therapies in Health and Medicine, 24*, 38–47.

through body movement. Ultimately, they find a new relationship to ease and discomfort, calm and agitation. As the individual finds a new relationship with the body—"trying on" new experiences—old habits tend to dissolve as more constructive ones are created.

Ethical inquiry becomes a part of this path for embodied realization as the person uses movement to experience qualities such as patience and kindness to facilitate joy or ease. The body becomes a mechanism for deeply understanding these new and positive experiences. Asana can be used as a transformative methodology to move abstract ethical qualities from mental construct to practical realization. The experience of ease or calm in the body brings a recognition of the reality of these concepts. Even when the mind resists, telling us that ease or calm is not possible, the body is teaching us that ease *is* possible, awakening an experience of hope and new possibilities. A home practice can be created to strengthen the new perceptual habit.

To serve as a transformative process, asana must be grounded in discriminative wisdom (differentiation between the body-mind-environment and essential nature as awareness); meaning and purpose; and ethical inquiry. As understood through this framework, yoga therapy may foster eudaimonic well-being and the qualities of spiritual well-being (see Figure 6.3). Through this lens, yoga therapy can affect health and well-being across the BPSS domains in various conditions and patient populations.

Conclusion

Clients usually come to healthcare professionals, including yoga therapists, with a primary concern—a "pain point" that they would like to understand and resolve. Any kosha or domain of health, or their combinations, may be the initiating factor prompting them to seek care. In addition, the initiating factor may differ from the concern the client currently reports. In other words, the reason the client comes to therapy may or may not be the initial factor that led to the dysfunction.

Under the BPSS and kosha models we explore each layer of experience and its contribution to pain, dysfunction, or suffering. The yoga therapy framework provides a holistic, systematic methodology through which we can assess these layers and guide clients in self-discovery that may include causes of dysfunction and intervention strategies in all domains of health and well-being.

Clinical Examples

Rotator Cuff Tendonitis

- *Physical domain/annamaya and pranamaya*
  Rotator cuff tendonitis is inflammation of one or more of the rotator cuff tendons of the shoulder. This condition often creates impingement and pain in the shoulder when the arm is lifted overhead. Patterns of tight or weak muscles around the shoulder develop as a result of pain and in turn perpetuate pain. Physical reasons for this dysfunction may be sustained postures (e.g., forward head carriage, rounded shoulders), prolonged time sitting at a computer or driving, or overuse injuries. Pain as well as any contributing postural dysfunction can alter breathing and movement patterns and produce an elevated stress response because of pain and loss

of function. The client may experience agitation, loss of vitality, or fatigue, which may further worsen the condition and heighten the experience of suffering.

- *Psychological domain/manomaya and vijnanamaya*
  Mental/emotional states can contribute to the posture and muscle imbalances responsible for rotator cuff impingement and tendonitis. Anxiety, stress, worry, or depression can create muscular tension that affects posture and movement of the shoulders. In other words, rather than a physical cause, muscular imbalances and dysfunction may be due to mental and emotional states. Mental and emotional states like worry may also result *from* the pain and loss of function associated with rotator cuff tendonitis. In other words, mental and emotional states may be both a cause and a result of physical dysfunction.

- *Social domain*
  Perceived social isolation can contribute to the pain and loss of function of physical problems, as perceived isolation affects inflammation, levels of disability, pain interference with activities, pain intensity, and mental/emotional states. Reciprocally, social isolation can become more pronounced as the person stops engaging in activity and experiences more disability, loss of meaningful relationships, and loneliness.

- *Spiritual domain/anandamaya*
  Diminished spiritual well-being can contribute to pain severity, intolerance, sensitivity, anxiety, depression symptoms, inflammation, and pain interference found with physical dysfunction. Inability to participate in previously meaningful activities can in turn create greater intrapersonal, relational, and existential disconnection.

The person may enter a physical therapy clinic with complaints of rotator cuff tendonitis, but the root cause is not the biomechanics of the shoulder. Rather, the cause of these holding patterns creating physical dysfunction may be mental or emotional concerns (anxiety, depression, grief); loneliness; or spiritual disconnection. A purely mechanical intervention to correct the musculoskeletal and fascial imbalances will be ineffective in the long term as long as these holding patterns persist.[13] No matter what manual therapies or exercises are provided, as long as the anxiety, perceived social isolation, or spiritual diminishment remains, the shoulder pain and rotator cuff impingement will return.

We can see the same cascading relationship from any portal of entry into the BPSS or kosha system.

Anxiety or Depression

- *Physical domain/annamaya and pranamaya*
  Patterns of tension in the body can reflect mental and emotional states. Depression or anxiety can create musculoskeletal imbalances such as tension or disconnects that limit function and create pain. These psychological states can also affect systemic physiological functions including those of the cardiovascular, nervous, gastrointestinal, and immune systems. Reciprocally, these physiological dysfunctions can worsen anxiety or depression symptoms. For example, autonomic dysregulation (e.g., heightened sympathetic "fight or flight" states) may produce either agitated states or fatigue, lethargy, or depressed states (see Chapter 7).
- *Psychological domain/manomaya and vijnanamaya*
  Patterns of thoughts, emotions, and beliefs about oneself, others, or life as well as traumatic events can contribute to anxiety or depression symptoms.
- *Social domain*
  Anxiety or depression may impede participation in activities and hinder the development of healthy, meaningful relationships. In turn, loneliness and perceived isolation may make it difficult for the person to participate in activities.
- *Spiritual domain/anandamaya*
  Anxiety or depression symptoms may promote feelings of intrapersonal, interpersonal, or existential disconnection and loss of meaning or purpose. Reciprocally, this disconnection and loss of meaning can worsen anxiety or depression symptoms.

No matter the doorway through which the suffering enters—physical, psychological, social, or spiritual—its effects ripple through each of the others, creating, for better or worse, an experience that encompasses all layers of being. A problem that starts in one domain affects the others. Through asana, pranayama, meditation, ethical inquiry, and more, yoga therapy seeks to address each domain synchronously to facilitate BPSS well-being.

Notes

1. King, M. B., & Koenig, H. G. (2009). Conceptualising spirituality for medical research and health service provision. *BMC Health Services Research*, 9(1). https://doi.org/10.1186/1472-6963-9-116; Koenig, H. G. (2012). Religion, spirituality, and health: The research and clinical implications. *ISRN Psychiatry*, 2012, 1–33; Koenig, H. G.,

130 Theoretical and Explanatory Frameworks

McCullough, M. E., & Larson, D. B. (2001). *Handbook of religion and health*. Oxford: Oxford University Press; Lysne, C. J., & Wachholtz, A. B. (2010). Pain, spirituality, and meaning making: What can we learn from the literature? *Religions, 2*(1), 1–16; Steinhauser, K. E., Fitchett, G., Handzo, G. F., Johnson, K. S., Koenig, H. G., Pargament, K. I., ... Balboni, T. A. (2017). State of the science of spirituality and palliative care research part I: Definitions, measurement, and outcomes. *Journal of Pain and Symptom Management, 54*(3), 428–440.

2. For some of the literature on this, see: Abbott, R. A., Martin, A. E., Newlove-Delgado, T. V., Bethel, A., Thompson-Coon, J., Whear, R., & Logan, S. (2017). Psychosocial interventions for recurrent abdominal pain in childhood. *The Cochrane Database of Systematic Reviews, 1*, CD010971. https://doi.org/10.1002/14651858.CD010971.pub2; Cacioppo, J. T., & Cacioppo, S. (2014). Social relationships and health: The toxic effects of perceived social isolation: Social relationships and health. *Social and Personality Psychology Compass, 8*(2), 58–72; Cacioppo, J. T., Hawkley, L. C., Norman, G. J., & Berntson, G. G. (2011). Social isolation. *Annals of the New York Academy of Sciences, 1231*(1), 17–22; Cole, S. W. (2013). Social regulation of human gene expression: Mechanisms and implications for public health. *American Journal of Public Health, 103*(S1), S84–S92; Eisenberger, N. I., Jarcho, J. M., Lieberman, M. D., & Naliboff, B. D. (2006). An experimental study of shared sensitivity to physical pain and social rejection. *Pain, 126*(1), 132–138; Evers, A. W., Kraaimaat, F. W., Geenen, R., Jacobs, J. W., & Bijlsma, J. W. (2003). Pain coping and social support as predictors of long-term functional disability and pain in early rheumatoid arthritis. *Behaviour Research and Therapy, 41*(11), 1295–1310; Karayannis, N. V., Baumann, I., Sturgeon, J. A., Melloh, M., & Mackey, S. C. (2019). The impact of social isolation on pain interference: A longitudinal study. *Annals of Behavioral Medicine, 53*(1), 65–74; López-Martínez, A. E., Esteve-Zarazaga, R., & Ramírez-Maestre, C. (2008). Perceived social support and coping responses are independent variables explaining pain adjustment among chronic pain patients. *Journal of Pain, 9*(4), 373–379; Norman, G. J., Hawkley, L., Ball, A., Berntson, G. G., & Cacioppo, J. T. (2013). Perceived social isolation moderates the relationship between early childhood trauma and pulse pressure in older adults. *International Journal of Psychophysiology, 88*(3), 334–338; Oliveira, V. C., Ferreira, M. L., Morso, L., Albert, H. B., Refshauge, K. M., & Ferreira, P. H. (2015). Patients' perceived level of social isolation affects the prognosis of low back pain: Social isolation and low back pain. *European Journal of Pain, 19*(4), 538–545; Ong, A. D., Uchino, B. N., & Wethington, E. (2016). Loneliness and health in older adults: A mini-review and synthesis. *Gerontology, 62*(4), 443–449.

3. Boyle, P. A., Barnes, L. L., Buchman, A. S., & Bennett, D. A. (2009). Purpose in life is associated with mortality among community-dwelling older persons. *Psychosomatic Medicine, 71*(5), 574–579; Cole, S. W., Levine, M. E., Arevalo, J. M. G., Ma, J., Weir, D. R., & Crimmins, E. M. (2015). Loneliness, eudaimonia, and the human conserved transcriptional response to adversity. *Psychoneuroendocrinology, 62*, 11–17; Dezutter, J., Casalin, S., Wachholtz, A., Luyckx, K., Hekking, J., & Vandewiele, W. (2013). Meaning in life: An important factor for the psychological well-being of chronically ill patients? *Rehabilitation Psychology, 58*(4), 334–341; Dezutter, J., Luyckx, K., & Wachholtz, A. (2015). Meaning in life in chronic pain patients over time: Associations with pain experience and psychological well-being. *Journal of Behavioral Medicine, 38*(2), 384–396; King & Koenig, Conceptualising spirituality for medical research and health service provision; Koenig, Religion, spirituality, and health; Koenig, McCullough, & Larson, *Handbook of religion and health*;

Krause, N. (2009). Meaning in life and mortality. *The Journals of Gerontology Series B: Psychological Sciences and Social Sciences, 64B*(4), 517–527; Lysne & Wachholtz, Pain, spirituality, and meaning making; Nsamenang, S. A., Hirsch, J. K., Topciu, R., Goodman, A. D., & Duberstein, P. R. (2016). The interrelations between spiritual well-being, pain interference and depressive symptoms in patients with multiple sclerosis. *Journal of Behavioral Medicine, 39*(2), 355–363; Ryff, C. D. (2014). Psychological well-being revisited: Advances in the science and practice of eudaimonia. *Psychotherapy and Psychosomatics, 83*(1), 10–28; Seybold, K. S. (2007). Physiological mechanisms involved in religiosity/spirituality and health. *Journal of Behavioral Medicine, 30*(4), 303–309; Wachholtz, A. B., & Pearce, M. J. (2009). Does spirituality as a coping mechanism help or hinder coping with chronic pain? *Current Pain and Headache Reports, 13*(2), 127–132; Wachholtz, A. B., Pearce, M. J., & Koenig, H. (2007). Exploring the relationship between spirituality, coping, and pain. *Journal of Behavioral Medicine, 30*(4), 311–318.
4. King & Koenig, Conceptualising spirituality for medical research and health service provision; Koenig, Religion, spirituality, and health; Vaillant, G. E. (2008). Positive emotions, spirituality and the practice of psychiatry. *Mens Sana Monographs, 6*(1), 48.
5. Cole et al., Loneliness, eudaimonia, and the human conserved transcriptional response to adversity.
6. Fredrickson, B. L., Grewen, K. M., Algoe, S. B., Firestine, A. M., Arevalo, J. M. G., Ma, J., & Cole, S. W. (2015). Psychological well-being and the human conserved transcriptional response to adversity. *PLOS ONE, 10*(3), e0121839. https://doi.org/10.1371/journal.pone.0121839
7. Fredrickson, B. L., Grewen, K. M., Coffey, K. A., Algoe, S. B., Firestine, A. M., Arevalo, J. M. G., … Cole, S. W. (2013). A functional genomic perspective on human well-being. *Proceedings of the National Academy of Sciences, 110*(33), 13684–13689; Fredrickson et al., Psychological well-being and the human conserved transcriptional response to adversity.
8. Ryff, C. D., Singer, B. H., & Dienberg Love, G. (2004). Positive health: Connecting well-being with biology. *Philosophical Transactions of the Royal Society B: Biological Sciences, 359*(1449), 1383–1394.
9. Ryff, Psychological well-being revisited.
10. Keyes, C. L., & Simoes, E. J. (2012). To flourish or not: Positive mental health and all-cause mortality. *American Journal of Public Health, 102*(11), 2164–2172.
11. Dezutter et al., Meaning in life; Dezutter, Luyckx, & Wachholtz, Meaning in life in chronic pain patients over time; Schleicher, H., Alonso, C., Shirtcliff, E. A., Muller, D., Loevinger, B. L., & Coe, C. L. (2005). In the face of pain: The relationship between psychological well-being and disability in women with fibromyalgia. *Psychotherapy and Psychosomatics, 74*(4), 231–239.
12. For more on the explanatory framework of yoga therapy, see Sullivan, M. B., Moonaz, S., Weber, K., Taylor, J. N., & Schmalzl, L. (2018). Toward an explanatory framework for yoga therapy informed by philosophical and ethical perspectives. *Alternative Therapies in Health and Medicine, 24*, 38–47.
13. Pain science literature is demonstrating the complex biopsychosocial-spiritual contributors to pain beyond the mechanistic. For more information, see N. Pearson, S. Prosko, & M. Sullivan. (2019). *Yoga and science in pain care: Treating the person in pain.* London: Singing Dragon.

Neurophysiological Perspectives

7

This chapter builds on the philosophical foundation introduced in Chapter 6, adding a neurophysiological perspective to the theoretical framework of yoga therapy. These neurophysiological concepts can help create a shared language between those in healthcare or research and yoga therapists.

Neurophysiological theories also add insight into possible applications of yogic practices to promote outcomes such as eudaimonic well-being and improved health across the biopsychosocial-spiritual domains. It is hoped that this work will help yoga to be understood in alignment with its philosophical context and provided in a manner that facilitates the practice's synergistic effects.

Salutogenesis and Pathogenesis: Complementary Perspectives for Health

The biomedical model described in Chapter 6 focuses largely on pathogenesis, investigation of the causes of disease or illness. Biomedical interventions address the contributors to a specific pathology, an approach well-suited to treat diseases that can be ascribed to a specific cause. A shortcoming of the pathogenic perspective becomes apparent when it is applied to complex or chronic conditions that involve more complex and/or less tangible factors (e.g., the social and spiritual factors discussed in Chapter 6).

Salutogenesis offers an alternative and complementary perspective to pathogenesis. Rather than focusing on the pathological cause of disease, the salutogenic model explores the origins of optimal states of health or well-being. Solely removing disease is not seen as sufficient to promote optimal function and thriving. Salutogenesis posits that well-being is more than the absence of disease. Salutogenic interventions focus on inclusive support of the factors that promote health.

It is important to note that the perspectives of pathogenesis and salutogenesis are not mutually exclusive and can complement each other in client care (see Table 7.1). The client can benefit from the pathogenic model for the prevention, removal, or lessening of pathology. At the same time, the salutogenic model supports clients along a continuum of care that promotes optimal health and well-being. Furthermore, salutogenic interventions can positively affect factors contributing to pathogenic states. When the models are used together, clients benefit from both the potential alleviation of pathology and greater well-being.

Ananda Balayogi Bhavanani teaches that yoga therapy is a salutogenic intervention.[1] This essential insight helps us to move away from *yogopathy*, where we apply yoga therapy through a biomedical, pathogenic lens focused on allopathic diagnoses and outcomes. Yoga therapy can be better

Table 7.1 Differences in Salutogenic and Pathogenic Paradigms

	Salutogenesis	*Pathogenesis*
Core question	What leads to health and well-being?	What leads to disease and pathology?
Aim	Identification of the factors that contribute to health	Identification of the factors that contribute to disease
Outcome sought	Optimal states of health and well-being, flourishing, improved quality of life	Removal of pathology or disease to support health
Purpose of interventions	To support and promote health and well-being (pathology may diminish in the process); possibility of improving states of health and well-being beyond the removal of disease	To support and promote the removal of disease for health to occur
Impact	Cultivates the potential for positive health through greater biopsychosocial-spiritual well-being	Diminishes the negative effect of pathology on health outcomes

understood through a salutogenic lens by which the practices and philosophy facilitate optimal states of well-being.

As a salutogenic intervention, yoga therapy can be incorporated into client care in various settings.

- **Acute care:** Yoga therapy can facilitate improved energy, sleep, mood, and emotional regulation, as well as decreased fatigue and stress. Each of these factors supports the effects of allopathic and pathogenic interventions and outcomes.
- **Chronic conditions:** Chronic conditions such as diabetes, rheumatoid arthritis (RA), and multiple sclerosis (MS) require long-term management and lifestyle support. Using RA as an example, yoga therapy can increase stability, strength, and mobility of the musculoskeletal system for greater function in daily life; improve sleep and energy levels for enhanced biopsychosocial-spiritual health; and decrease stress and allostatic load (see p. 136) to help regulate inflammation and nervous system and endocrine function.
- **Enhancing community:** As mentioned in Chapter 6, social support has profound effects for physical and mental health outcomes and can improve long-term disease management. Yoga classes that meet the specific needs of a population—for example, stroke survivors—can build social support and connection. I have been part of both hospital programs and independent organizations offering this kind of outreach to groups with chronic conditions such as pain, cancer, and traumatic brain injury.
- **Hospice and end-of-life care:** Yoga therapy in these settings supports greater ease, meaning, and contentment. Rather than prolonging life, yoga therapy can help people cultivate such qualities as connection, insight, and peace.
- **The "well" population:** Yoga therapy promotes optimal states of well-being for those in good health, potentially preventing pathological states and encouraging greater functioning.

To summarize, pathogenic interventions can diminish disease states, whereas salutogenic interventions can positively affect disease states and promote optimal health or well-being. Incorporating a salutogenic perspective is vital to a more comprehensive approach to client care. Rather than solely focusing on the alleviation of disease, we can also support flourishing and address the contribution of social and spiritual factors to physical and mental health.

Fostering Salutogenesis

Homeostasis and Allostasis

Homeostasis and allostasis are important concepts in the idea of salutogenic intervention for health and well-being. Although the meaning of these terms continues to evolve, a few basics can further understanding of the neurophysiological underpinnings of salutogenic interventions like yoga therapy.

Homeostasis can be defined as the maintenance of vital body systems (e.g., pH, temperature, glucose levels) within a limited range for survival. In the face of challenging, stressful, or threatening circumstances homeostasis preserves these essential aspects of physiological function.[2]

Although the human system works to maintain its systems within an optimal range, life naturally entails stressors that challenge homeostatic processes. Far from being entirely negative, the experience of stress enables us to develop a more flexible, adaptive system that responds to situations appropriately. As such, it is crucial for our bodies to learn how to navigate these stressors and processes of change

We can consider stress responses on a continuum. On one end, stressors can lead to healthy systemic adaptation. On the other end, the system may become overwhelmed, leading to adverse health effects. In unhealthy responses to stress, we are unable to maintain stability in our systems as we meet environmental demands. Either prolonged exposure to stressful events or momentary traumatic situations can overwhelm the system. In both cases, the inability to maintain homeostasis results in excessive exposure to the mediators of the stress response. This situation can damage the body through depletion of resources, breakdown of systems, or wear and tear.[3]

Allostasis and *allostatic load* explain the adverse effects of unhealthy stress. Allostasis means to maintain stability through change, which helps an organism to adjust to both predictable and unpredictable circumstances.[4] It describes the dynamic processes that maintain stability of our vital systems in response to both predictable and unpredictable stressors or events, even to the point of possible detriment to other systems. As the demands of life challenge homeostasis, allostasis stabilizes the body's essential systems for survival. Allostatic processes maintain key markers amidst adverse or stressful situations. In other words, as we respond to stressors through a mobilization response (i.e., increased heart rate, blood pressure, cortisol levels, and muscle tension), survival systems, such as those that regulate pH, glucose, and body temperature, are maintained.

The term allostasis brings nuance to the concept of stress, differentiating between the systems that need to be stabilized for life (homeostasis) and the processes that maintain that stability in the face of challenge, change, or adversity (allostasis). The dynamic processes of allostasis support homeostasis.

Allostasis fosters homeostasis through mediators that include hormones, neurotransmitters, and cytokines. The "stress response" mediators of the hypothalamic-pituitary-adrenal (HPA) axis and sympathetic nervous system are crucial to this function of allostasis (see Definitions, p. 136). Allostatic processes and mediators like the stress response are beneficial and adaptive in the short term as they stabilize the system, helping us to gain flexibility and strength in response to challenge. However, the meditators of allostasis can become detrimental if they overwhelm the system or remain elevated for sustained periods.

Allostatic load indicates this "cumulative cost to the body of allostasis."[5] This term helps to describe the damage to the body that results from the wear and tear of prolonged exposure to allostatic states, which can predispose us to injury or disease. Chronic hypertension or elevation of inflammatory cytokines, for example, contributes to the development of pathological conditions including atherosclerotic plaques, neuronal remodeling or loss, chronic pain, impaired immunity, obesity, and bone demineralization.[6] It is important to understand that the nuances of stress include a continuum from healthy adaptation in response to changing stimuli to unhealthy overload that damages systems. Allostasis and allostatic load help to explain how protective and healthy mediators of stress can have unhealthy consequences.

Definitions

Allostasis: dynamic processes that help an organism maintain stability of its vital systems in response to both predictable and unpredictable stressors or events, even to the point of possible detriment to these and other systems.

Allostatic load: cumulative cost to the body of engaging in allostatic processes over a prolonged period.

Autonomic nervous system (ANS): branch of the nervous system that monitors and influences the level of activation of many body systems including the cardiovascular, endocrine, respiratory, digestive, immune, and musculoskeletal systems. Functions such as heart rate, blood pressure, respiration, intestinal motility and digestion, and muscular tone are all under the control of the ANS. The sympathetic and parasympathetic nervous systems are two branches of the ANS.

Homeostasis: the maintenance of vital systems within the limited range required for survival.

Parasympathetic nervous system (PNS): branch of the autonomic nervous system responsible for restoration of the system. PNS activation provides the conditions for optimal healing, growth, and conservation of resources. Commonly referred to as the *rest and digest response* or *relaxation response,* PNS activation is essential to homeostasis.

Stress response: in response to perceived danger or threat, the body mobilizes for action via activation of the sympathetic branch of the ANS. In addition, the endocrine system is involved through activation of the hypothalamic-pituitary-adrenal (HPA) axis. The stress response includes increased muscle tone, heart rate, and respiratory rate; release of hormones such as catecholamine; and inhibited gastrointestinal function to free up resources for the mobilization of the system toward safety.

Sympathetic nervous system (SNS): branch of the autonomic nervous system responsible for the mobilization of body systems (e.g., cardiovascular, respiratory, endocrine) to meet any demand. SNS activation includes any response to real or perceived dangers or stressors in both the internal and external environments. It is commonly referred to as the *fight-flight-freeze response* or *stress response.*

Promoting Regulation and Resilience

The conscious ability to manage or alter responses to threat, challenge, or adversity for homeostasis is termed *self-regulation*. Self-regulation depends on the ability to recognize and influence thoughts, emotions, behavior, and physiological states. We can foster both physical and psychological well-being by attending to body and mind states, as well as by cultivating the capacity to change these states in response to stimuli.

The capacity to regulate body-mind reactions to stress is linked to decreased allostatic load. Learning self-regulatory skills can help us conserve resources and maintain or return to healthier states in response to physiological, psychological, or environmental challenge. Through this effect on allostatic load, self-regulation is considered an important contributor to improved health and well-being in conditions such as irritable bowel syndrome, anxiety, neurodegenerative disorders, trauma, depression, and chronic pain.[7]

Resilience is related to self-regulation and allostasis, adding a component of the efficiency with which we recover from stress or adversity. A resilient system recovers quickly, conserving physical and psychological resources.[8] Measures of resilience include both levels of physiological activation and psychological attitudes, behaviors, and emotions in response to stimuli. Chronic stress, adversity, and sustained allostatic load can compromise resilience. Higher resilience has been linked to many positive health outcomes, including less perceived stress, greater motivation in recovery from illness or trauma, better adjustment to serious diagnoses, and better management of chronic pain.[9]

Mind-Body Practices: Top-Down and Bottom-Up Strategies for Regulation and Resilience

Mind-body practices such as yoga are thought to help improve regulation and resilience and to decrease allostatic load through their integrated effects on physiological and emotional states and on behavior.[10] These practices may facilitate bidirectional communication between the body and mind in response to potential or actual challenge. This communication is commonly referred to as top-down neurocognitive and bottom-up neurophysiological processes. Mind-body practices are proposed to benefit various patient populations through this framework.[11]

Top-down neurocognitive processes involve various types of mental practice or focus, including intentional practices such as compassion meditation or application of the ethical principles of yoga (yama and niyama). The term *top-down* denotes the cascading effects of these cognitively based practices, through which thought, emotion, and belief influence physiological states and behavior. These "thought-based" practices help us regulate attention and set specific intentions toward mind states like peace, calm, or equanimity. Top-down processes result in coordinated regulation of systems including the nervous, endocrine, cardiovascular, and immune systems.[12]

Cardiologist and mind-body professor Herbert Benson's *relaxation response*[13] describes the effect of a top-down practice. Mental focus activates the parasympathetic nervous system (PNS), countering sympathetic activity and mitigating allostatic load (see Definitions, p. 136). The repetition of a word, phrase, or image creates this integrated response through the physiological systems of relaxation. The relaxation response includes decreased heart rate, blood pressure, "stress hormones" such as cortisol, and inflammation, as well as improved immunity and digestive motility.

In addition to prompting physiological change, top-down practices of visualization or focus can affect behavior and one's relationship to others. Through visualizing a peaceful place, repeating a phrase like "I am filled with peace," or practicing loving-kindness we may gain insight into a different way of approaching life circumstances. If our habitual reaction to a stressful situation or person is anger or anxiousness, for example, the practice of compassion or loving-kindness may help us pause in our reactions to consider other perspectives and responses, regulate the body and mind to a calm state, and respond in healthier, more adaptive ways.

Bottom-up processes are initiated in the body and create a cascade of effects whereby change in physiological state alters psychological state and behavior. Breath practices and movement can affect bodily systems such as the cardiovascular, nervous, musculoskeletal, and digestive systems. These changes can then influence perception, emotion, cognition, and behavior.[14]

Practices such as lengthening the exhale or engaging alternate-nostril breathing can activate the relaxation response with its many systemic effects to mitigate allostatic load. In addition to this active regulation offered by breath practices, research points to links among respiratory pattern, autonomic nervous system state, and emotion. Emotions—sadness, happiness, anger, fear—are associated with distinct respiratory patterns and autonomic nervous system (ANS) states as measured by heart rate and heart rate variability (HRV) (see Understanding Vagal Control, p. 140).[15]

Breath regulation is a powerful tool to offer a client. Pranayama techniques teach us that we have the power to access a parasympathetic state even under stressful circumstances, and we come to understand the link between emotional state and breath pattern. Breathing practices help us develop a sense of self-efficacy as we recognize the potential to regulate our systems and to create healthier, more adaptive responses both physically and psychologically.

We can also initiate bottom-up processes through movement, body position, or physical exercise. Movement of the body directly affects physiological systems such as the cardiorespiratory and nervous systems. In addition, specific movements have been associated with emotions: Rising, expansive, light, rhythmic, jumping movements are predictive of happiness; sinking, passive weight, and head-down postures are predictive of sadness; enclosing, condensing, backward, and retreating movements are predictive of fear; and advancing, sudden movements and direct effort are predictive of anger.[16]

Both breath and movement offer powerful tools for self-regulation and resilience. Through them we can learn that we have the capacity to shift to a parasympathetic state and to cultivate the relaxation response. We can also uncover the relationships among autonomic state, respiratory pattern, and emotional characteristics.

Understanding Vagal Control

Heart rate variability (HRV), more specifically respiratory sinus arrhythmia, is often used as a measure of vagal control or regulation. HRV reflects the natural fluctuations in heart rate that happen during respiration in a parasympathetic state, when vagal influence is dominant. In this resting state, the heart rate naturally increases on the inhale and decreases on the exhale. In a sympathetically dominant state, this variability decreases or disappears.

Greater vagal regulation of the heart, which is measured through respiratory sinus arrhythmia (shown by high-frequency HRV), is correlated with greater stress resilience and flexibility to respond to challenges; improved interoception; improved emotional and attentional regulation; and differential activation in brain regions that regulate responses to threat appraisal.[17]

Lower vagal regulation of the heart, measured as low HRV, has been correlated with chronic conditions such as fibromyalgia; musculoskeletal pain conditions such as low back, neck, shoulder, and pelvic pain; IBS; headaches; and rheumatoid arthritis (RA). In addition, low HRV is also associated with poor self-regulation, less behavioral flexibility, and adverse health outcomes such as increased mortality in lupus, RA, and trauma.[18]

It is important to note that these studies are looking at the impact of parasympathetic state on the heart for health and well-being. This gives important information on the relationship between parasympathetic cardiac control and well-being but does not necessarily provide a clinical picture of systemic parasympathetic state and how it affects overall health and well-being. An evaluation of whole-person parasympathetic state would include other systems besides cardiac control—peripheral circulation, cortisol levels, and blood pressure, to name a few. To assess the full function of the social engagement system, as discussed under "Polyvagal Theory" (see p. 149), Porges and his lab measure vagal regulation of the heart, affect recognition, auditory processing dependent on middle ear function, and vocal prosody.

HRV has been used to demonstrate yoga's ability to improve autonomic regulation through parasympathetic cardiac activation. Understanding yoga's effect on vagal regulation can assist in translating its effects for broad-based promotion of physical, mental, and behavioral health. Through the mechanism of improved vagal control, yoga can help to create greater well-being and salutogenesis in various conditions such as neurodegenerative diseases, cancers, cardiovascular problems, and PTSD. Put another way, through an integration of top-down and bottom-up practices, yoga influences the vagus nerve to promote self-regulation and systemic physiological, psychological, and behavioral health.

The Importance of Bottom-Up Processes

Meditation, intention-setting, and other top-down cognitively based practices are powerful, but they are not always accessible or appropriate. Clients may resist these suggestions or feel that the cognitive practices are forced or fake, particularly when they are overwhelmed by sadness, anger, or fear. In such cases, bottom-up processes use the body as an entry point for accessing and influencing physiological and emotional states and behavioral attributes that might not otherwise be approachable.

The body's tangibility helps us experience different perceptions. A change in physical position can prompt discovery of emotional states or behavioral attributes that may have previously seemed unavailable. Creating a palpable experience of these different states challenges long-held beliefs, making the body a gateway for transformation. Ultimately, we learn that there are many options for responding and relating to the body, mind, and life.

The potential for body position and movement to foster different physiological and emotional states makes yoga postures a powerful tool for transformation and for building self-regulatory skills and resilience. We can use this knowledge in our implementation of asana, for example, using gentle rhythmic motion or positions of expansion like sidebending or supported backbending to facilitate experiences such as happiness or contentment.

In my own clinical practice, I have often found the truth of this idea that the body can teach something the mind resists. When one's mind does not allow for an experience, the body can serve as a powerful means to challenge beliefs that may be perpetuating patterns of pain or suffering. For example, someone with chronic pain may not believe that the absence of pain is possible, or someone with anxiety may not believe that calm or contentment is possible. Physical movement and postures can support experiences through which to discover these new possibilities. For example, a client I worked with thought of herself as weak, fearful, and lacking confidence. She had difficulty feeling as if she could navigate the stressors of life. Mountain, warrior, and bridge postures enabled her to feel strength and surety. As she experienced her body in this new way, she both challenged her habitual beliefs and created new potential, discovering her inherent strength and confidence to meet life differently.

I think of this process as creating a template, or blueprint, of a different state through the body. The body becomes a laboratory where we can "try on" different experiences, a particularly useful method when someone is overwhelmed by an emotional experience or long-held belief. We can experiment with postures that provide an opposing state to the habitual one, exploring body positions that bring an experience of openness, lightness, happiness, or connection. This process empowers clients to recognize that they have access to a diverse array of perspectives, beliefs, and behaviors. Once these experiences have been templated, the client can return to the posture to reinforce the availability of this full spectrum of possibility for relating to themselves and the world. The body teaches the mind—and the whole person—what the mind cannot arrive at through cognitive processes alone.

Yoga Therapy to Catalyze Top-Down and Bottom-Up Processes

A framework for yoga suggests that this integration of top-down (yama/niyama and meditation) and bottom-up (asana, pranayama) practices fosters systemic body-mind regulation and mitigates allostatic load to benefit diverse client populations such as those with depression, post-traumatic stress disorder (PTSD), and chronic pain.[19] Research has corroborated yoga's capacity to facilitate physical and mental regulation and resilience as well as its integrated effects on autonomic function, emotion, and attention.[20]

Chapter 6 described the framework of yoga therapy through the lens of eudaimonic and social/spiritual well-being. This chapter defines translational neurophysiological language to benefit healthcare and research contexts. The teachings of yoga provide a systematic methodology for integrating the practices of ethics, meditation, physical postures, and breathwork. Through a neurophysiological and psychological lens, this theoretical framework can be understood as the facilitation of salutogenesis by promoting body-mind regulation and resilience and decreasing allostatic load. We can expect that the practices' effects will be enhanced when implemented synergistically within this framework.

A translational language can help those less familiar with yoga view the practice through its own theoretical framework. As a result, yoga therapy can be understood as a complementary and integrative healthcare profession with distinct benefits for client care in diverse populations.

The Autonomic Nervous System

The ANS is a key mediator of salutogenesis (see Definitions, p. 136). The ANS monitors and influences the level of activation of many body systems including the cardiovascular, endocrine, respiratory, digestive, immune, and musculoskeletal systems. These connections to the various functions make the ANS essential for decreasing allostatic load, improving systemic regulation and resilience, and for communication between the body and the brain. Functions such as heart rate, blood pressure, respiration, intestinal motility and digestion, and muscular tone are all under the control of the ANS. Through this system our hearts pump blood, we breathe, and digestion occurs without us having to consciously remember to do so.

Because of its extensive reach, the ANS plays a crucial role in assessing, controlling, and responding to internal and external stimuli in an integrated way. The ANS is responsible for creating a unified systemic response to cues of potential threat or safety through a continuum of mobilization and restoration.

Often, the ANS is described dichotomously, with an antagonistic relationship between the parasympathetic and sympathetic responses (see Definitions, p. 136). The parasympathetic nervous system (PNS) is portrayed as countering the mobilization of the sympathetic nervous system (SNS) to promote restoration. This view of opposition is inaccurate as it does not consider the vast array of interactions that are possible in response to stimuli. Our organs often receive input from both branches of the ANS, resulting in a range of potential responses. The ANS can employ this spectrum of control—from co-activation of the SNS and PNS to withdrawal or increase of their activity—over any organ.[21]

Let's consider the heart as an example to illustrate this variable influence of the ANS to fine-tune our responses to any circumstance. In a relaxed state, the heart is under parasympathetic control through the vagus nerve. When a stimulus to mobilize the system is perceived, the ANS helps to create an increase in heart rate. Initially, the vagus nerve decreases its influence on the heart, which increases the heart rate. This first stage of mobilization is not due to sympathetic activation, but rather represents a release of parasympathetic control, a "lifting off" of PNS restraint. If this increase in heart rate is not enough to meet the demands of the situation, the sympathetic system will exert its influence to increase the heart rate even more.

These diverse possibilities for activation translate to wide variability in how the ANS affects the body's systems in any moment and in response to stimuli. In sum, the SNS and PNS cooperate to create a variety of strategies to efficiently meet environmental demands.

Neuroception and the Initiation of Autonomic States

Neuroception, a term coined by behavioral neuroscientist and creator of polyvagal theory Stephen Porges, is the subconscious detection of environmental safety or danger influencing underlying ANS activation.[22] Neuroception occurs before conscious interpretation by higher brain centers and includes the perception of both inner bodily state and the external environment. An integrated physiological, emotional, and behavioral response is then established through ANS activation, ideally generating a quick and efficient response to perceived danger or safety.

The autonomic state activated by neuroception becomes a *neural platform* from which combined physiological, emotional, and behavioral attributes emerge.[23] For example, perceiving threat may activate the neural platform of the SNS, or fight-flight-freeze. As a result, we experience physiological mobilization as well as emotional and behavioral attributes (e.g., anger, fear, anxiety) that enable us to respond quickly to the perceived danger. Through neuroception, information from the inner and the outer world is perceived, the degree of safety or threat is assessed, and an autonomic response influencing physiology, emotion, and behavior is generated.

Polyvagal theory, developed by Porges, describes three neural platforms and five global states that can be produced by this subconscious detection of safety or danger.[24] Each platform and state is associated with particular and related physiological, emotional, and behavioral attributes, as discussed later in the chapter.

Understanding these neural platforms and the process of neuroception is important to the discussion of regulation of the body, mind, and behavior for optimal health and well-being. Mind-body practices, including yoga, teach us to become more aware of our autonomic state and the stimuli that activate certain neural platforms, bringing conscious attention to our subconscious reactions. Such insight can help us learn self-regulatory skills so that we respond to internal and external stimuli in healthier ways. For example, when you enter a room, your five senses take in the colors of the walls, smells in the air, people and objects, and so on. This sensory information, *exteroception,* is combined with internal bodily sensation such as digestive processes, cardiovascular functions, and respiratory rate to create a feeling of safety or danger. Through the process of neuroception, these stimuli activate autonomic neural platforms through which certain emotions, feelings, and behaviors arise or become likely (see Figure 7.1). Misclassifying a situation may produce inappropriate or unhealthy activations—we may react to safe situations as though dangerous and vice versa.

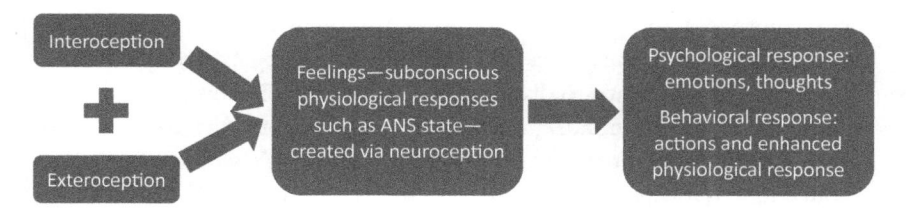

Figure 7.1 A Neurophysiological Description of Discriminative Wisdom in Yoga.

Note: Information enters the body-mind via exteroception (input from the five senses) and interoception (viscera and internal bodily state), creating a feeling. *Feeling* here refers to the felt sense of subconscious physiological experience as a result of interoceptive and exteroceptive input and could include such descriptors as heavy, light, withered, full, agitated, or calm. In addition to feelings, or as a contributor to these feelings, subconscious neurophysiological states become activated. Neuroception is part of this response, as it represents the ANS state set up by the combined interoceptive and exteroceptive inputs to help us prepare for appropriate physical and emotional responses. From the feelings and subconscious activations of neurophysiological state, emotions and actions arise to foster safety, regulation, and homeostatic balance.

Yoga helps us to become more conscious of these habitual subconscious reactions so we can consciously choose more adaptive responses to our environment.

Interoception: Sensing Internal State—and More

Historically, *interoception* was defined as the perception of sensory visceral information. However, its meaning has become more complex over time to include emotion, cognition, memory, as well as the integration of and response to information. Current conceptual understandings of interoception include the afferent sensory pathways within the body and viscera that convey information to brain structures; the receipt, interpretation, and integration of that information; the pathways that enact a response to the information and help maintain homeostasis; and our emotional and cognitive perceptions.[25] Distinct characteristics of interoception are now being defined and include interoceptive awareness (noticing inner stimuli like heartbeat), sensitivity (minimum threshold for detecting signals), and accuracy (ability to discriminate among signals).[26]

The concept of interoception is helpful in exploring the relationships between emotional and physiological signals as well as our response to and integration of such signals with thoughts, beliefs, and memories. Importantly, for our purposes, interoception is a translatory neurophysiological concept that describes part of the process of discrimination in yoga. Through discriminative wisdom, we learn to distinguish between the phenomena of prakriti (stimuli of the body, mind, and environment) and purusha to clarify the causes of suffering and recognize our essential nature as awareness.

Building interoceptive skills enables us to become aware of how we sense, interpret, and process physiological, emotional, and environmental stimuli. Moreover, the relationships between physiological sensation, cognitive/emotional experience, and environmental stimuli become apparent. Insight develops as we become more proficient at identifying what is arising in the body, mind, and environment as well as how these signals relate to one another. Improved interoception helps us acquire healthier, more appropriate responses for improved homeostatic balance, self-regulation, and resilience.[27] In addition, this skill supports the establishment of discriminative wisdom in yoga, which enables intentional life choices.

Figure 7.1 represents a way I have taught clients and students about the cultivation of discriminative wisdom in yoga in terms of these neurophysiological concepts. This schema is adapted from the work of a number of researchers.[28]

Clinical Relevance

We can teach clients to move backward through the process shown in Figure 7.1, starting from noticing behaviors and emotions to considering underlying feelings, systemic activations, and ultimately interoceptive and exteroceptive input. Eventually, the client is able to identify and discern the stimuli that shape their feelings, emotions, and actions. For example, via interoception and exteroception we may have a felt sense of agitation in our chest and our ANS may activate a sympathetic neural platform in response to perceived or actual threat. We interpret these physiological states emotionally and behaviorally. Actions such as muscular tension as well as emotions such as anger or fear may emerge to facilitate movement toward safety.

The person learns to disentangle each response component—actions, emotions, feelings, neurophysiological activations, interoceptive stimuli, exteroceptive stimuli—clarifying their influence on emotion and behavior. They come to understand how feelings and perceptions can be interpreted as emotions and acted on through behavior. This learning can help the person to inquire into any of these components to better understand them.

Someone who has recurrent back pain may notice that the pain arises alongside emotions (e.g., sadness, anxiety, anger); neurophysiological activations (e.g., sympathetic states); feelings (e.g., fatigue, stress, agitation, heaviness); or exteroceptive input (e.g., a person or situation). As observational powers strengthen, connections among physiological states, emotions, and pain may become apparent. We can then teach the client to be aware of the signals or situations that precipitate their pain. When they first notice these signals, even before or at the beginning of pain, they can employ yogic techniques to alter their responses and mitigate pain.

Yoga therapy has many tools to help with this process. Practices can help clients to nonjudgmentally observe and explore the relationships between the perception of inner and outer stimuli (interoception and exteroception) and feelings, neurophysiological activations, emotions, and behavior. As the capacity for observation becomes stronger, movement, breath, and meditation can be employed to change reactions to each response component to decrease suffering or pain. Through both top-down neurocognitive and bottom-up neurophysiological practices, yoga changes our emotional and behavioral reactions and relationships to interoceptive and exteroceptive input, feelings, and neurophysiological activations. This improved sensitivity promotes systemic regulation and salutogenesis. (Practices that foster interoceptive skills are the focus of Chapter 10.)

A Deeper Look at ANS Regulation

The ANS affects physiological, emotional, and behavioral states, so its regulation is key to systemic health and overall well-being. Regulation of the ANS indicates balanced and appropriate activation of the PNS and SNS in response to inner and outer stimuli. A well-regulated and resilient system is one that responds optimally to challenges and efficiently returns to a homeostatic state for healing and restoration.

When the ANS is dysregulated, excessive or insufficient SNS or PNS activity may result. A dysregulated system is one that is less adaptable and flexible in response to stimuli. Autonomic dysregulation may lead to various adverse health effects, contribute to allostatic load, and diminish systemic resilience. Imbalance of the ANS places the body under constant stress, challenging homeostasis. As ANS dysregulation is often present in chronic conditions, it is proposed to play a role as an effect of the condition, a contributor to its development, or both.[29]

Chronic conditions, including pain, create constant stress on the body, leading to ANS dysregulation and allostatic load. Conversely, ANS dysregulation itself contributes to allostatic load and diminishes resilience, worsening the condition. Conditions that involve ANS dysregulation and are helped by promoting ANS regulation and resilience include irritable bowel syndrome (IBS), neurodegenerative disorders, chronic pain, anxiety, depression, RA, headaches, and fibromyalgia.[30]

A Detailed Look at the Vagus Nerve

A deeper understanding of the vagus nerve is essential as we dive into more complex theories of the ANS and its capacity to promote systemic regulation and resilience. The vagus nerve is the 10th cranial nerve, and its name means *wandering*—fitting for a structure that begins in the brainstem and branches out to communicate with viscera such as the heart, lungs, and intestines. As a *mixed nerve,* the vagus carries information both toward and away from the central nervous system. The vagus is a bidirectional conduit of information between the body (visceral and somatic tissues) and the brain.

The vagus is composed of about 80% sensory, or *afferent,* fibers. This means that it carries information, such as visceral state, from the periphery to the central nervous system structures of the spinal cord and brain. With its widespread branches, the sensory component of the vagus is a key conveyer of interoceptive information about the state and function of the body to the brain. The vagus is also key to neuroception and the initiation of autonomic activations in response to perceived danger or safety.

The rest of the vagus nerve's fibers, about 20%, are motor, or *efferent*. In its motor role, the vagus nerve is a major supporter of parasympathetic states (including those influenced by heart rate, respiration, inflammation, muscular tone, and digestion) that promote systemic homeostasis, restoration, and growth.

Significantly, polyvagal theory describes two separate origination sites of the motor vagus nerve from different nuclei in the brainstem—the dorsal motor nucleus and the nucleus ambiguus. These two source nuclei form separate motor branches of the vagus and help to explain the diverse continuum of parasympathetic responses to perceived danger or safety. Rather than a system solely for resting and digesting, the PNS can create a range of effects, as detailed below.[31]

Several additional important functions of the vagus nerve are relevant to our discussions.[32] Vagal afferents are essential to both interoception and neuroception, as they bring information from the body to the brainstem and higher brain structures. This information is processed through the hypothalamus, which is responsible for regulation of ANS activity. Because these nerve branches from the vagus communicate with higher brain centers, they influence sensory and motor integration, pain modulation, memory, attention, and emotional regulation.[33]

Its multifactorial influence has made the vagus a focus of research exploring autonomic function and its relationship to connected physiological and emotional states and behavior.[34] The vagus nerve is thought to have a unique role in the mind–body system with its widespread connections to viscera, internal structures, the brainstem, and higher brain structures. This broad network, and the nerve's dual motor and sensory functions, place the vagus in a crucial role as a link between both body and mind states and behavior.

In sum, the vagus is responsible for providing information about bodily states to the brain and functions as a mediator of systemic regulation and resilience by promoting parasympathetic states. The capacity to influence underlying autonomic state through vagally mediated pathways is significant for health and well-being. By affecting both the relationship to interoceptive information as well as underlying autonomic activations we can shape our experience of and response to physical, emotional, and environmental stimuli.

Polyvagal Theory: Connected and Emergent Physiological, Emotional, and Behavioral Characteristics

Polyvagal theory offers a complex, dynamic understanding of the ANS.[35] The theory describes foundational autonomic neural platforms from which shared physiological, emotional, and behavioral attributes emerge. The primary neural platforms, which comprise three of the five global states, are described below. These states are based on varying levels of activation of the SNS, the motor branch of the vagus nerve from the nucleus ambiguus, and the motor branch of the vagus nerve from the dorsal motor nucleus. Co-activation of these three platforms results in the other two global states. Both interoception and neuroception are important to the establishment of these autonomic states.

Primary Neural Platforms

Social Engagement System

The neural platform of social engagement describes the activation arising from a network of nerves including the nucleus ambiguus branch of the vagus nerve, the motor components of the glossopharyngeal nerve, spinal accessory nerve, trigeminal nerve, and facial nerve. The vagal branch involved in this motor response—stemming from the nucleus ambiguus—is responsible for the production of respiratory sinus arrhythmia, the measure of HRV used to demonstrate parasympathetic dominance and a resting state of the heart (see Understanding Vagal Control, p. 140).

The social engagement platform is activated in response to perceived safety in the environment and results in:

- physiological restoration and homeostasis, including slowed heart and respiratory rates, greater HRV, and improved peristalsis for digestion;
- activation of the muscles of facial expression, creating greater calm, safety, and understanding between individuals;
- attunement to the human voice, enabling better distinction of human sounds from surrounding noise; and
- control of the muscles of the throat, producing improved vocal prosody (i.e., the ability to fine-tune speech to be more pleasing or relaxing to others).

The synergistic activation of these nerves links the muscles of the face, inner ear, and throat with a resting state of the heart for coordinated control. This neural platform is termed the *social engagement system* because a restorative, homeostatic bodily state is coupled with greater likelihood of interpersonal connection through both receptive (hearing) and expressive (vocal prosody and facial expression) domains of communication. A resting physical state and greater capacity for connection with others increase the likelihood that positive emotional states and prosocial behavioral attributes—compassion, love, equanimity, eudaimonic well-being—will emerge.[36]

The social engagement system is activated in response to a neuroception of safety based on interoceptive and exteroceptive stimuli. As this neural platform promotes positive physical, emotional, and behavioral states it is essential to the concepts of regulation and salutogenesis.

The top-down and bottom-up processes initiated through yogic practices strengthen the capacity to activate the neural platform of social engagement. In addition, the discernment cultivated through yoga brings conscious attention to the subconscious perceptions and reactions of neuroception. We can learn to regulate our systems and gain facility in returning to the social engagement state more quickly and efficiently after stress, creating greater resilience. (Chapter 9 focuses on practices that cultivate these skills.)

Defensive Mobilization, or SNS Dominance

The *defensive mobilization* neural platform is the fight-flight response represented by activation of the SNS. This defensive strategy of mobilization occurs in response to perceived threat in the environment and includes increased muscle tone, heart rate, and respiratory rate; release of hormones such as catecholamine (related to stress); and inhibited gastrointestinal function. In addition to orienting the body toward mobilization for survival, the brain is activated toward attention and response to potential threat. As a result of this shift in physiological state, emotions like fear, anger, or anxiety may emerge, reflecting the need to find protection. As a response to perceived threat or danger, a combined physiological, attentional, emotional, and behavioral state mobilizes the system to safety.

Defensive Immobilization

The neural platform of *defensive immobilization* is thought to be activated in response to extreme threat, danger, or terror. Engagement of this platform results in a dramatic slowing of the body's processes to the minimum necessary for survival. Defensive immobilization diminishes heart rate, muscle tone, and all bodily systems to the lowest possible energy output. The branch of the vagus nerve originating in the brainstem's dorsal motor nucleus is thought to be largely responsible for this response. This neural platform, referred to as the *death-feigning response,* is the most passive response to stressful situations. As a response to a perception of extreme threat, a combined physiological state of immobilization or shutdown is connected with emotional or behavioral states that might include disembodied or dissociative attributes.

During the Bhagavad Gita's pivotal pre-battle moment, when Arjuna collapsed on the field at Kurukshetra, we can suppose that his ANS was in a state of defensive immobilization—he may even have been experiencing the shutdown of an extreme dorsal-vagal response.

Co-Activated States

The neural platforms of social engagement, defensive mobilization, and defensive immobilization produce a range of autonomic responses from restoration to mobilization to shutting down, respectively. Polyvagal theory also describes a range of parasympathetic responses from optimal homeostatic, relaxed, and connected states (social engagement) to a dramatic slowing down and immobilization of the system (defensive immobilization). To add to the complexity, these three neural platforms are not isolated, either/or situations. Rather, they comingle to create the vast array of possible human behavior and experience. Two final global states arise from the interaction of the three foundational neural platforms.

Safe Mobilization

The global state of *safe mobilization* represents co-activation of the neural platforms of social engagement and the SNS (defensive mobilization). It is present in situations, such as play, dance, exercise, and creative endeavors, in which the system is mobilized for action but safety is perceived. The social engagement neural platform provides a foundation for positive emotional and prosocial qualities, while the sympathetic neural platform enables mobilization for action to meet healthy demands. The result is a simultaneous neuroception of safety and mobilization through which we can experience connection while the bodymind is mobilized for movement and quick thinking.

The concept of safe mobilization is key in helping to promote regulation and, even more so, resilience. We can learn to find safety, calm, and restoration within a mobilized system, creating a larger container—wider tolerance—for life's stressors. As a result, we meet stimuli without becoming overwhelmed by activation of the body or mind. This skill is key in moving toward optimized salutogenesis. In other words, learning to co-activate the neural platforms of social engagement and defensive mobilization enables us to manage stressors more effectively and efficiently, resulting in less allostatic load on the system and therefore better physical and mental health.

Yogic practices are well-suited to teach the capacity for safe mobilization. For example, attentional or meditation techniques such as intention-setting, visualization, and breath control can initiate the social engagement neural platform while working in active postures, as detailed in Chapter 11. We can then experience mobilization of the body's resources with a calm state of mind or easy respiration, and the resulting larger container of safe activation can be mirrored in life situations.

Safe Immobilization

Safe immobilization represents co-activation of the social engagement neural platform (stemming from the nucleus ambiguus branch of the vagus) and the defensive immobilization neural platform (stemming from the dorsal motor nucleus branch of the vagus). This global state is theorized to be present with simultaneous perception of safety and dorsal motor nucleus activation that immobilizes the system or slows metabolic resources. Safe immobilization, in which we maintain safety and social connection alongside stillness, occurs in situations such as states of meditation and relaxation. It is also proposed to occur in childbirth, orgasm, and nursing.[37]

Conclusion

Polyvagal theory helps to illuminate the connections among physiology, emotion, and behavior resulting from underlying ANS activations. Learning to shift these neural platforms may simultaneously promote greater physical, mental, and behavioral health through improved regulation and resilience.

Practices that initiate the social engagement neural platform lay the foundation for self-regulation by promoting healthy homeostatic physiological states, positive psychological states (e.g., calm, contentment), and prosocial behavioral states (e.g., compassion). Eudaimonic well-being, with its widespread effects for physical and mental health, may also be fostered by this activation.

The neural platforms of safe mobilization and safe immobilization promote resilience through practices that activate the SNS or states of stillness, respectively, concurrent with an anchor of calm provided by control of the breath or attention. Ultimately, such experiences foster safe activation and wider tolerance of stimuli, enabling us to better navigate whatever arises in the body, mind, or environment.

Autonomic dysfunction, with its far-reaching physical, psychological, and behavioral effects, is often described as a contributor to, or cause of, many conditions, including cardiovascular, immune, metabolic, musculoskeletal, trauma, and pain disorders. Conversely, promoting regulation and resilience through autonomic control facilitates greater physical, psychological, and behavioral health and well-being in populations with these conditions. By learning to shift autonomic state with yoga therapy practices, we can initiate concurrent effects on physiology (including muscle tone, heart rate, stress-hormone release, and gastrointestinal function), emotional states, and behavior. Unlike a pathology-oriented practice, yoga therapy can be understood as an integrated salutogenic practice that facilitates top-down and bottom-up processes for autonomic regulation and resilience.

Applying yoga therapy as a cohesive system rather than isolated practices fosters healthy autonomic states. When integrated, tools such as yama, niyama, meditation, asana, and pranayama affect underlying neural platforms for healthy physiology, emotion, and behavior. With an intention of facilitating the social engagement neural platform, yoga therapy encourages states such as eudaimonic well-being, compassion, and connection. The practices can also be oriented toward the neural platforms of safe mobilization and safe immobilization for greater systemic resilience.

Notes

1. Bhavanani, A. B. (2011). Are we practicing yoga therapy or yogopathy? *Yoga Therapy Today*, 7(2), 26–28; Bhavanani, A. B., Sullivan, M., Taylor, M. J., & Wheeler, A. (2019). Shared foundations for practice: The language of yoga therapy. *Yoga Therapy Today*, Summer, 44–47.
2. For more on homeostasis, see: McEwen, B. S. (2005). Stressed or stressed out: What is the difference? *Journal of Psychiatry and Neuroscience*, 30(5), 315; McEwen, B. S., & Wingfield, J. C. (2003). The concept of allostasis in biology and biomedicine. *Hormones and Behavior*, 43(1), 2–15.
3. McEwen, Stressed or stressed out; McEwen & Wingfield, The concept of allostasis in biology and biomedicine.
4. For more on allostasis and allostatic load, see McEwen & Wingfield, The concept of allostasis in biology and biomedicine.
5. McEwen & Wingfield, The concept of allostasis in biology and biomedicine, p. 12.
6. McEwen, Stressed or stressed out; McEwen & Wingfield, The concept of allostasis in biology and biomedicine.
7. Muehsam, D., Lutgendorf, S., Mills, P. J., Rickhi, B., Chevalier, G., Bat, N., ... Gurfein, B. (2017). The embodied mind: A review on functional genomic and neurological correlates of mind–body therapies. *Neuroscience & Biobehavioral Reviews*, 73, 165–181; Schmalzl, L., Powers, C., & Henje Blom, E. (2015). Neurophysiological and neurocognitive mechanisms underlying the effects of yoga-based practices: Towards a comprehensive theoretical framework. *Frontiers in Human Neuroscience*, 9. https://doi.org/10.3389/fnhum.2015.00235; Streeter, C. C., Gerbarg, P. L., Saper, R. B., Ciraulo, D. A., & Brown, R. P. (2012). Effects of yoga on the autonomic nervous system, gamma-aminobutyric-acid, and allostasis in epilepsy, depression, and post-traumatic stress disorder. *Medical Hypotheses*, 78(5), 571–579; Taylor, A. G., Goehler, L. E., Galper, D. I., Innes, K. E., & Bourguignon, C. (2010). Top-down and bottom-up mechanisms in mind-body medicine: Development of an integrative framework for psychophysiological research. *EXPLORE: The Journal of Science and Healing*, 6(1), 29–41.

8. Tugade, M. M., & Fredrickson, B. L. (2004). Resilient individuals use positive emotions to bounce back from negative emotional experiences. *Journal of Personality and Social Psychology, 86*(2), 320–333; Whitson, H. E., Duan-Porter, W., Schmader, K. E., Morey, M. C., Cohen, H. J., & Colón-Emeric, C. S. (2016). Physical resilience in older adults: Systematic review and development of an emerging construct. *The Journals of Gerontology Series A: Biological Sciences and Medical Sciences, 71*(4), 489–495.
9. Resnick, B., Galik, E., Dorsey, S., Scheve, A., & Gutkin, S. (2011). Reliability and validity testing of the physical resilience measure. *The Gerontologist, 51*(5), 643–652.
10. Taylor, Goehler, Galper, Innes, & Bourguignon, Top-down and bottom-up mechanisms in mind-body medicine.
11. Schmalzl, Powers, & Henje Blom, Neurophysiological and neurocognitive mechanisms underlying the effects of yoga-based practices; Taylor, Goehler, Galper, Innes, & Bourguignon, Top-down and bottom-up mechanisms in mind-body medicine; Gard, T., Noggle, J. J., Park, C. L., Vago, D. R., & Wilson, A. (2014). Potential self-regulatory mechanisms of yoga for psychological health. *Frontiers in Human Neuroscience, 8*. https://doi.org/10.3389/fnhum.2014.00770
12. Muehsam et al., The embodied mind; Taylor, Goehler, Galper, Innes, & Bourguignon, Top-down and bottom-up mechanisms in mind-body medicine.
13. Benson, H., & Klipper, M. Z. (2000). *The relaxation response*. New York: HarperTorch.
14. Muehsam et al., The embodied mind; Taylor, Goehler, Galper, Innes, & Bourguignon, Top-down and bottom-up mechanisms in mind-body medicine.
15. Rainville, P., Bechara, A., Naqvi, N., & Damasio, A. R. (2006). Basic emotions are associated with distinct patterns of cardiorespiratory activity. *International Journal of Psychophysiology, 61*(1), 5–18.
16. Shafir, T., Tsachor, R. P., & Welch, K. B. (2016). Emotion regulation through movement: Unique sets of movement characteristics are associated with and enhance basic emotions. *Frontiers in Psychology, 6*. https://doi.org/10.3389/fpsyg.2015.02030
17. Adlan, A. M., Veldhuijzen van Zanten, J. J. C. S., Lip, G. Y. H., Paton, J. F. R., Kitas, G. D., & Fisher, J. P. (2017). Cardiovascular autonomic regulation, inflammation and pain in rheumatoid arthritis. *Autonomic Neuroscience, 208*, 137–145; Park & Thayer, From the heart to the mind; Porges, *The polyvagal theory: Neurophysiological foundations of emotions, attachment, communication, and self-regulation*; Streeter, Gerbarg, Saper, Ciraulo, & Brown, Effects of yoga on the autonomic nervous system.
18. Adlan et al., Cardiovascular autonomic regulation, inflammation and pain in rheumatoid arthritis; Azam, Katz, Mohabir, & Ritvo, Individuals with tension and migraine headaches exhibit increased heart rate variability during post-stress mindfulness meditation practice; Barakat et al., Dysregulation of the autonomic nervous system is associated with pain intensity; Caceres, C., & Burns, J. W. (1997). Cardiovascular reactivity to psychological stress may enhance subsequent pain sensitivity. *PAIN, 69*(3), 237–244; Koenig et al., Pneumogastric (vagus) nerve activity indexed by heart rate variability in chronic pain patients compared to healthy control; Meeus et al., Heart rate variability in patients with fibromyalgia and patients with chronic fatigue syndrome; Park & Thayer, From the heart to the mind; Sowder, E., Gevirtz, R., Shapiro, W., & Ebert, C. (2010). Restoration of vagal tone: A possible mechanism for functional abdominal pain. *Applied Psychophysiology and Biofeedback, 35*(3), 199–206; Staud, Heart rate variability as a biomarker of fibromyalgia syndrome; Tsuji, H., Venditti, F. J., Manders, E. S., Evans, J. C., Larson, M. G., Feldman, C. L., & Levy, D. (1994). Reduced heart rate

variability and mortality risk in an elderly cohort. The Framingham Heart Study. *Circulation, 90*(2), 878–883.
19. Schmalzl, Powers, & Henje Blom, Neurophysiological and neurocognitive mechanisms underlying the effects of yoga-based practices; Gard, Noggle, Park, Vago, & Wilson, Potential self-regulatory mechanisms of yoga for psychological health; Streeter, Gerbang, Saper, Ciraulo, & Brown, Effects of yoga on the autonomic nervous system.
20. Chu, I.-H., Wu, W.-L., Lin, I.-M., Chang, Y.-K., Lin, Y.-J., & Yang, P.-C. (2017). Effects of yoga on heart rate variability and depressive symptoms in women: A randomized controlled trial. *Journal of Alternative and Complementary Medicine, 23*(4), 310–316; Dale, L. P., Carroll, L. E., Galen, G. C., Schein, R., Bliss, A., Mattison, A. M., & Neace, W. P. (2011). Yoga practice may buffer the deleterious effects of abuse on women's self-concept and dysfunctional coping. *Journal of Aggression, Maltreatment & Trauma, 20*(1), 90–102; Mackenzie, M. J., Carlson, L. E., Paskevich, D. M., Ekkekakis, P., Wurz, A. J., Wytsma, K., … Culos-Reed, S. N. (2014). Associations between attention, affect and cardiac activity in a single yoga session for female cancer survivors: An enactive neurophenomenology-based approach. *Consciousness and Cognition, 27*, 129–146; Sarang, P., & Telles, S. (2006). Effects of two yoga based relaxation techniques on heart rate variability (HRV). *International Journal of Stress Management, 13*(4), 460–475; Telles, S., Sharma, S. K., Gupta, R. K., Bhardwaj, A. K., & Balkrishna, A. (2016). Heart rate variability in chronic low back pain patients randomized to yoga or standard care. *BMC Complementary and Alternative Medicine, 16*(1). https://doi.org/10.1186/s12906-016-1271-1; Tyagi, A., & Cohen, M. (2016). Yoga and heart rate variability: A comprehensive review of the literature. *International Journal of Yoga, 9*(2), 97. https://doi.org/10.4103/0973-6131.183712
21. Paton, J. F. R., Boscan, P., Pickering, A. E., & Nalivaiko, E. (2005). The yin and yang of cardiac autonomic control: Vago-sympathetic interactions revisited. *Brain Research Reviews, 49*(3), 555–565.
22. Porges, S. W. (2003). The polyvagal theory: Phylogenetic contributions to social behavior. *Physiology & Behavior, 79*(3), 503–513; Porges, S. W. (2004). Neuroception: A subconscious system for detecting threats and safety. *Zero to Three, 24*(5), 19–24; Porges, S. W. (2011). *The polyvagal theory: Neurophysiological foundations of emotions, attachment, communication, and self-regulation* (1st ed.). New York: W. W. Norton.
23. Porges, The polyvagal theory: Phylogenetic contributions to social behavior; Porges, *The polyvagal theory: Neurophysiological foundations of emotions, attachment, communication, and self-regulation*.
24. For more on polyvagal theory, see Porges, *The polyvagal theory: Neurophysiological foundations of emotions, attachment, communication, and self-regulation*.
25. Ceunen, E., Vlaeyen, J. W. S., & Van Diest, I. (2016). On the origin of interoception. *Frontiers in Psychology, 7*. https://doi.org/10.3389/fpsyg.2016.00743; Craig, A. D. (2015). *How do you feel?: An interoceptive moment with your neurobiological self*. Princeton, NJ: Princeton University Press; Porges, *The polyvagal theory: Neurophysiological foundations of emotions, attachment, communication, and self-regulation*.
26. Ceunen, Vlaeyen, & Van Diest, On the origin of interoception; Farb, N., Daubenmier, J., Price, C. J., Gard, T., Kerr, C., Dunn, B. D., … Mehling, W. E. (2015). Interoception, contemplative practice, and health. *Frontiers in Psychology, 6*. https://doi.org/10.3389/fpsyg.2015.00763

27. Farb et al., Interoception, contemplative practice, and health; Haase, L., Stewart, J. L., Youssef, B., May, A. C., Isakovic, S., Simmons, A. N., ... Paulus, M. P. (2016). When the brain does not adequately feel the body: Links between low resilience and interoception. *Biological Psychology, 113*, 37–45.
28. Damasio, A., & Carvalho, G. B. (2013). The nature of feelings: Evolutionary and neurobiological origins. *Nature Reviews—Neuroscience, 14*(2), 143–152; Craig, How do you feel?; Porges, *The polyvagal theory: Neurophysiological foundations of emotions, attachment, communication, and self-regulation*; Farb et al., Interoception, contemplative practice, and health.
29. Koenig, J., Falvay, D., Clamor, A., Wagner, J., Jarczok, M. N., Ellis, R. J., ... Thayer, J. F. (2016). Pneumogastric (vagus) nerve activity indexed by heart rate variability in chronic pain patients compared to healthy controls: A systematic review and meta-analysis. *Pain Physician, 19*(1), E55–78.; Kolacz, J., & Porges, S. W. (2018). Chronic diffuse pain and functional gastrointestinal disorders after traumatic stress: Pathophysiology through a polyvagal perspective. *Frontiers in Medicine, 5*. https://doi.org/10.3389/fmed.2018.00145; Streeter, Gerbarg, Saper, Ciraulo, & Brown, Effects of yoga on the autonomic nervous system; Tracy, L. M., Ioannou, L., Baker, K. S., Gibson, S. J., Georgiou-Karistianis, N., & Giummarra, M. J. (2016). Meta-analytic evidence for decreased heart rate variability in chronic pain implicating parasympathetic nervous system dysregulation. *PAIN, 157*(1), 7–29.
30. For examples of references, see: Azam, M. A., Katz, J., Mohabir, V., & Ritvo, P. (2016). Individuals with tension and migraine headaches exhibit increased heart rate variability during post-stress mindfulness meditation practice but a decrease during a post-stress control condition—A randomized, controlled experiment. *International Journal of Psychophysiology, 110*, 66–74; Barakat, A., Vogelzangs, N., Licht, C. M. M., Geenen, R., Macfarlane, G. J., de Geus, E., ... Dekker, J. (2012). Dysregulation of the autonomic nervous system is associated with pain intensity, not with the presence of chronic widespread pain. *Arthritis Care & Research, 64*(8), 1209–1216; Cohen, H., Neumann, L., Shore, M., Amir, M., Cassuto, Y., & Buskila, D. (2000). Autonomic dysfunction in patients with fibromyalgia: Application of power spectral analysis of heart rate variability. *Seminars in Arthritis and Rheumatism, 29*(4), 217–227; Kolacz & Porges, Chronic diffuse pain and functional gastrointestinal disorders after traumatic stress; Meeus, M., Goubert, D., De Backer, F., Struyf, F., Hermans, L., Coppieters, I., ... Calders, P. (2013). Heart rate variability in patients with fibromyalgia and patients with chronic fatigue syndrome: A systematic review. *Seminars in Arthritis and Rheumatism, 43*(2), 279–287; Muehsam et al., The embodied mind; Schmalzl, Powers, & Henje Blom, Neurophysiological and neurocognitive mechanisms underlying the effects of yoga-based practices; Staud, R. (2008). Heart rate variability as a biomarker of fibromyalgia syndrome. *Future Rheumatology, 3*(5), 475–483; Streeter, Gerbarg, Saper, Ciraulo, & Brown, Effects of yoga on the autonomic nervous system; Taylor, Goehler, Galper, Innes, & Bourguignon, Top-down and bottom-up mechanisms in mind-body medicine; Tracy et al., Meta-analytic evidence for decreased heart rate variability in chronic pain.
31. Porges, *The polyvagal theory: Neurophysiological foundations of emotions, attachment, communication, and self-regulation*.
32. For more on these convergences and vagal function in pain, see Erb, M., & Sullivan, M. (2019). Polyvagal theory and the gunas: A model for autonomic regulation in pain.

In N. Pearson, S. Prosko, & M. Sullivan (Eds.), *Yoga and science in pain care: Treating the person in pain*. London: Singing Dragon.
33. Frangos, E., Richards, E. A., & Bushnell, M. C. (2017). Do the psychological effects of vagus nerve stimulation partially mediate vagal pain modulation? *Neurobiology of Pain, 1*, 37–45; Park, G., & Thayer, J. F. (2014). From the heart to the mind: Cardiac vagal tone modulates top-down and bottom-up visual perception and attention to emotional stimuli. *Frontiers in Psychology, 5*. https://doi.org/10.3389/fpsyg.2014.00278
34. Porges, *The polyvagal theory: Neurophysiological foundations of emotions, attachment, communication, and self-regulation*; Porges, S. W. (2017). *The Oxford handbook of compassion science* (E. Seppala, Ed.). New York, NY: Oxford University Press.
35. For more on polyvagal theory and clinical applications, I recommend two books: Porges, *The polyvagal theory: Neurophysiological foundations of emotions, attachment, communication, and self-regulation* and Porges S., & Dana, D. (2018). *Clinical applications of the polyvagal theory: The emergence of polyvagal-informed therapies*. New York: W. W. Norton.
36. Pearson, Prosko, & Sullivan, *Yoga and science in pain care*; Porges, S. W., & Carter, C. S. (2017). Polyvagal theory and the social engagement system: Neurophysiological bridge between connectedness and health. In P. L. Gerbarg, P. R. Muskin, R. P. Brown (Eds.), *Complementary and integrative treatments in psychiatric practice* (pp. 221–240). Arlington, VA: American Psychiatric Association Publishing; Porges, *The polyvagal theory: Neurophysiological foundations of emotions, attachment, communication, and self-regulation*; Porges, *The Oxford handbook of compassion science*; Sullivan, M. B., Erb, M., Schmalzl, L., Moonaz, S., Noggle Taylor, J., & Porges, S. W. (2018). Yoga therapy and polyvagal theory: The convergence of traditional wisdom and contemporary neuroscience for self-regulation and resilience. *Frontiers in Human Neuroscience, 12*. https://doi.org/10.3389/fnhum.2018.00067
37. Kolacz & Porges, Chronic diffuse pain and functional gastrointestinal disorders after traumatic stress; Porges, *The polyvagal theory: Neurophysiological foundations of emotions, attachment, communication, and self-regulation*.

From Conceptual to Practical Application

Biomedical and Yogic Perspectives on Yoga Therapy

8

As described so far in this book, yoga therapy is a salutogenic intervention aimed at helping individuals alleviate suffering and foster well-being. Its practices can help us to flourish within our particular circumstances along a continuum from relative health and seeking greater function to acute situations, long-term chronic disease management, and end-of-life care. In each instance, the practices of yoga are adapted to the individual to support optimal well-being across the biopsychosocial-spiritual (BPSS) domains of health. This framework can be described from both yogic and healthcare/research perspectives starting with broad, conceptual understandings and moving to specific practical applications (see Figure 8.1).

Yogic and Psychophysiological Perspectives

Broad, Conceptual Understanding

Yoga supports a process of realization that encourages a sense of connectedness extending from oneself to others and the transcendent or existential. From a realization of connectedness, we may experience inner and outer harmony and equanimity, even amidst pain or suffering. Yoga's ethical practices of yama and niyama provide insight into actions and behaviors that further this harmony, meaning-making, and a purposeful life for the actualization of dharma.

In psychophysiological terms, yoga therapy can be said to promote overall well-being through a focus on spiritual and eudaimonic well-being. This

160 Theoretical and Explanatory Frameworks

Alleviation of Suffering/Salutogenesis

Broad/conceptual → Specific/practical

Language of Healthcare and Research (Psychophysiological Perspective)

- Eudaimonic and spiritual well-being
  - Personal, interpersonal, existential connection
  - Meaning and purpose
  - Virtue ethics
  - Self-realization/self-actualization/authenticity
- Biopsychosocial-spiritual well-being
  Systemic body-mind regulation and resilience
  - Neural platforms/autonomic nervous system effects
  - Interoceptive skill-building
- Initiation of top-down and bottom-up processes through the practices of yoga

Language of Yoga

- Realization of awareness
  - Connectedness extending from personal and interpersonal to transcendent/existential
  - Inner and outer harmony, or dharma/contentment/equanimity
  - Ethical practices
- Koshas
  - Prana vayus
  - Discernment between awareness, purusha, and prakriti
  - Gunas, aspects of "mind" and senses
  - Kleshas
- Yogic practices
  - Yama and niyama
  - Meditation
  - Asana
  - Pranayama

Broad/conceptual → Specific/practical

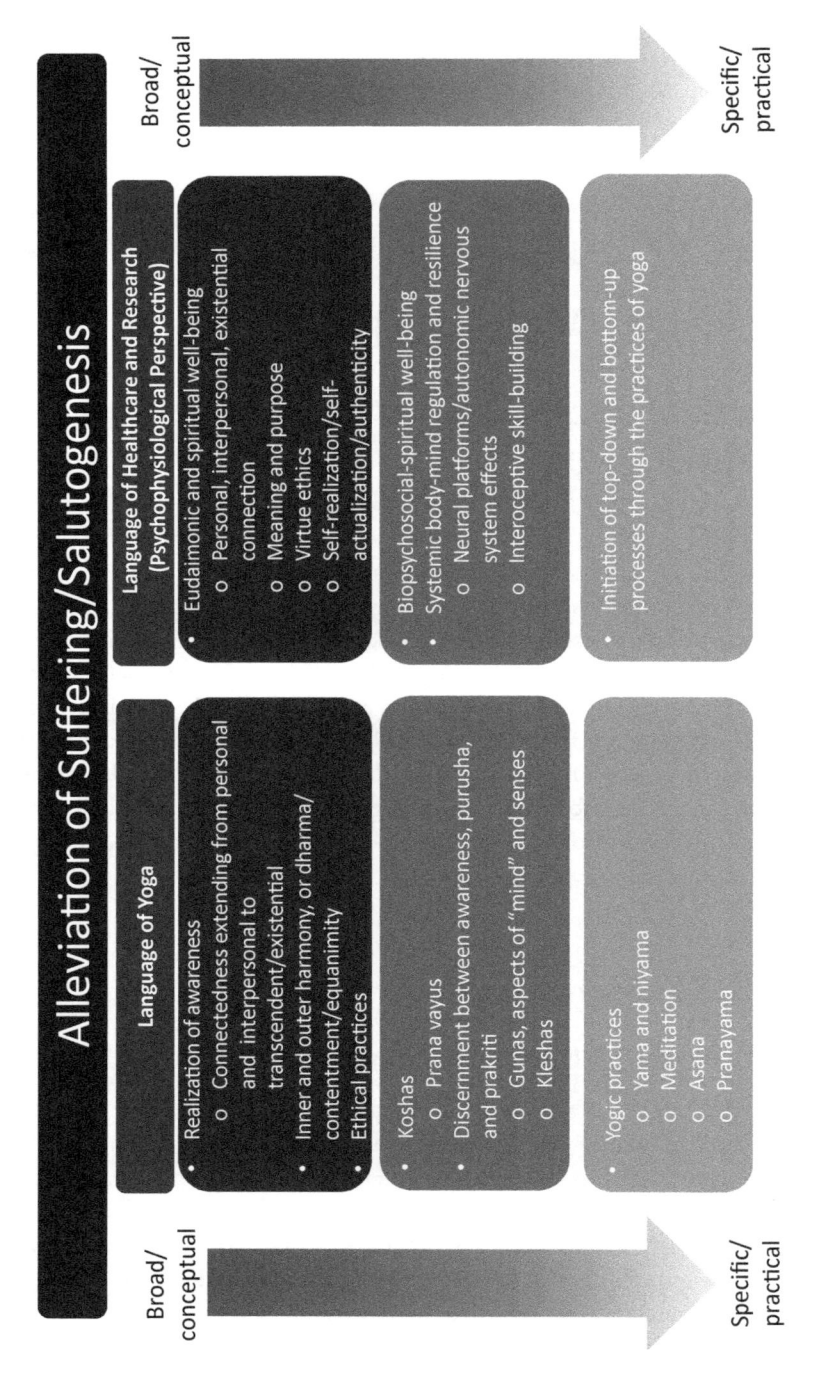

Figure 8.1 Yoga Therapy's Framework Can Be Described From Both Yogic and Psychophysiological Perspectives.

emphasis on connectedness, meaning and purpose, ethics, self-realization, and self-actualization supports healthy relationships with oneself, others, and life circumstances.

Toward Specificity

Yoga philosophy offers many avenues to understanding both the obstacles to and facilitators of well-being. One such teaching is the koshas, which help us to recognize that our experience is made up of layers from gross to subtle. Constructs like the prana vayus enable deeper inquiry into the more subtle and ambiguous layer of energy, or pranamaya.

Another philosophical tradition, samkhya, provides a systematic methodology for discerning fluctuating stimuli from awareness. This work includes developing an understanding of the gunas as the qualities of clarity, activity, and stillness that constitute all body-mind-environmental phenomena. Additionally, these aspects of the mind and senses serve as pathways of inquiry for discernment and realization. The Yoga Sutras of Patanjali teach the kleshas as an additional means of examining the obstacles that perpetuate our suffering.

In healthcare and research terminology, the BPSS model of integrative health provides an analogous model to the koshas for examining how the layers of experience affect one another.

Systemic body-mind regulation and resilience relate to discriminative wisdom in yoga as we learn to recognize and develop healthy relationships to body-mind-environmental stimuli. The neural platforms and global states of polyvagal theory, and their convergence with the gunas (detailed below), offer insight into the interconnected habits of body, mind, and behavior that improve or detract from health and well-being.

Interoception is essential for exploring the connections among bodily sensations, emotions, thoughts, beliefs, and behavior.[1] Interoceptive skills are thought to be important in pain and addiction, as these abilities help us interpret and respond to stimuli more accurately and appropriately in support of body-mind self-regulation and resilience.[2] Through discriminative wisdom as well as insight into subtle-body concepts such as prana and the prana vayus, yoga can foster healthy interoceptive skills for systemic (body-mind) regulation and resilience.

Eudaimonic and spiritual well-being become the overarching framework through which discernment, regulation, and resilience promote BPSS health and well-being.

Yoga and Psychophysiological Perspectives on Regulation and Resilience

Neural Platforms of Polyvagal Theory and Gunas of Yoga

Convergences between the neural platforms of polyvagal theory and the gunas of yoga enable the translation of yoga therapy, based on its wisdom tradition, into current contexts. Both models provide an insightful framework for understanding connections among bodily states, mental processes, and behavior as well as systemic regulation and resilience. I have explained this framework, as outlined below, with colleagues including Stephen Porges.[3]

The neural platforms of polyvagal theory and the gunas of yoga are foundations from which interconnected physiological, emotional, and behavioral states emerge. From the particular combination and predominance of neural platforms or gunas, these related states manifest. Altering the activation of the neural platform or guna can change the body, mind, and behavior in widespread and concurrent ways.

The gunas and neural platforms have reciprocal relationships—when one is activated, its counterpart is likely to manifest. In other words, each guna is reflected in a corresponding neural platform and vice versa as they support and reinforce one another.

Under the influence of any of the gunas a particular neural platform is likely to manifest (see Table 8.1):

- Sattva guna predominance supports attributes of clarity, lightness, and calm, which encourages activation of the social engagement neural platform with its parasympathetic response and positive psychological and prosocial attributes.
- Predominance of raja guna, with its influence to mobilize, supports activation of the neural platforms of safe mobilization and defensive mobilization, encouraging a continuum of mobilization from creativity and play to anger, anxiety, or fear.
- Tama guna predominance supports states of stillness or solidity, which encourages activation of the neural platform of safe immobilization or defensive immobilization. This effect spans a continuum of stillness from stability, groundedness, or intimacy to obscuration, dissociation, death-feigning, or inertia.

The same relationships can be understood from the perspective of neural platforms. When a neural platform is activated, certain gunas with shared attributes are likely to emerge or become predominant. For example, activating the social engagement system, with its attributes of calm and connection, encourages the predominance of sattva guna; activating the neural platforms of mobilization (safe or defensive mobilization) encourages raja guna; and activating the neural platforms of immobilization (safe or defensive immobilization) encourages tama guna.

Sattva and the Social Engagement System: Substrates for Regulation

Sattva guna and the social engagement neural platform both reflect regulated states that support BPSS well-being. These conditions include physical

Table 8.1 Convergent Properties of the Gunas and Neural Platforms

Neural Platform/ Global State	Guna (Yogic Philosophy)	Shared Physiological, Emotional, and Behavioral Characteristics
Social engagement: predominant activation of ventral vagal complex	Predominance of sattva	Safety, connection, illumination, lucidity, compassion, relaxation, calm
Safe mobilization: co-activation of ventral vagal complex and sympathetic nervous system	Balance of sattva with rajas	Activity, creativity, motivation, capacity for change, capacity for being active and alert yet relaxed (e.g., play or dance)
Defensive mobilization: predominant activation of sympathetic nervous system	Predominance of rajas	Fear, anger, greed, agitation, anxiety, tension, activation of physiological systems for fight-flight responses
Safe immobilization: co-activation of dorsal vagal complex and ventral vagal complex	Balance of sattva with tamas	States of progressive deep relaxation or meditation, stillness, stability, groundedness, intimacy, social bonding
Defensive immobilization: predominant activation of dorsal vagal complex	Predominance of tamas	Obscuration, inertia, dullness, ignorance, delusion, dissociation, hypotonia, slowing of physiological systems for conservation of resources to the lowest output needed for survival

restoration and homeostasis; mental and emotional qualities such as calm, equanimity, and contentment; and prosocial behaviors like compassion and connectedness.

The neural platform of social engagement cultivates these characteristics through its effects on facial expressivity, hearing, and vocal prosody. The parasympathetic activation that is part of this neural platform also produces relaxed, calm, restorative physiological states. Similarly, a predominance of sattva guna promotes body-mind states of tranquility, contentment, and the recognition of connection among all beings. From the clarity of sattva, we gain insight into our true nature as awareness with its concomitant attributes of steadfast joy, contentment, and equanimity.

Healthier connection to one's own body and mind is supported by the properties of sattva guna and the social engagement neural platform. The calm and clarity possible here provide the capacity for the nonjudgmental, compassionate observation essential for the development of discriminative wisdom. The establishment of equanimity helps us to explore reactions to stimuli, and to build the interoceptive skills necessary for healthy and adaptive relationships to physical and mental sensations. Greater interpersonal and existential connections are also found in sattva guna and social engagement, where qualities such as compassion, patience, and generosity support the creation of better relationships, meaning-making in adverse situations, and living a purposeful life. Inner and outer harmony between one's own values and actions in life are supported by discernment, interoceptive awareness, meaning-making, and inner/outer connectedness.

When situated in sattva guna or the social engagement neural platform, we learn to identify strategies that encourage mental, emotional, and physical regulation including the cultivation of restoration. Relaxed body-mind states and the capacity to self-regulate are keys to salutogenesis and improved BPSS health and well-being. By engaging in practices that strengthen sattva guna we can activate the social engagement neural platform; likewise, by activating the social engagement neural platform we encourage the emergence of sattva guna.

We can orient yogic practices to promote this activation. Ethical inquiry and meditation can be used to foster loving-kindness, nonharming, compassion, connectedness, as well as parasympathetic activations. Breath techniques and movement/postures that facilitate a parasympathetic state and support experiences of joy, calm, or connection may also encourage the activation of the social engagement neural platform and sattva guna. These practices, the focus of Chapter 9, provide a starting point for initiating systemic regulation for physical and mental health.

Rajas, Tamas, and Changing Neural Platforms: Substrates for Resilience

Although sattva provides an important foundational experience, the goal of yoga is not to be situated in sattva 100% of the time. Life naturally consists of the fluctuations of the gunas. Through the experiences of rajas, tamas, and sattva we are able to discern material nature from awareness and realize states of eudaimonic well-being. It is thus imperative, and a goal of yoga, to learn how to navigate these qualities so that we understand ourselves and our world and can decrease suffering.

The emergent properties of rajas and tamas share similarities with the neural platforms for mobilization and immobilization, respectively. When these gunas are balanced with sattva guna, they produce healthy levels of creativity (rajas) and stability (tamas). Similarly, when the social engagement platform is co-activated with the platforms of mobilization or immobilization, play, creativity, stillness, bonding, and intimacy emerge.

When rajas or tamas predominate, they can overpower the clarity of sattva to create agitation, anxiety, obscuration, inertia, and dullness. Correspondingly, activation of defensive mobilization or defensive immobilization can suppress the social engagement system. A perception of danger subverts the calm, connected states of social engagement.

Resilience is a key aspect of the importance of learning to navigate the fluctuations of the gunas and neural platforms. Chapter 7 introduced resilience as the capacity to respond adequately to stressors and to efficiently return to a restorative state. A healthy individual is one who can fine-tune his responses to stressors along a continuum of possible activations and restorations as appropriate to the situation.

Yoga teaches the capacity for resilience through recognition that the movement of the gunas is inherent to life. Richard Miller describes the lifespan of everything that comprises material nature, including the physical body itself, as an evolving cycle: Every thought, emotion, belief, bodily sensation, and worldly event is born, grows, matures, diminishes, and decays. The neural platforms reflect these fluctuations as their activations shift in response to circumstances such as perceived threat or safety and factors such as hunger, fatigue, or thoughts.

We cannot escape the fluctuations of material nature, including the gunas and the neural platforms. No person is ever free of this movement, which will happen even if we try to stop it. To not embrace this reality is to shut off from life, which makes us susceptible to spiritual bypassing (see Chapter 3). The teachings of yoga do not ask us to ignore or isolate ourselves from life, but rather to experience and change our relationship with it. Being clear and present with all that life presents enables us to be resilient and to respond to each situation to our fullest potential. This complete attention to what is being offered in each moment is the heart of resilience.

To learn resilience, yoga teaches us how to recognize the movement of the gunas, strengthen sattva as a foundation, and ultimately navigate the movement of the gunas. By learning to be patient, allow stillness, and find contentment and connection within, we can become present to the lifespan of each phenomenon. We learn to nonjudgmentally observe and experience the movement of the gunas without *becoming* them. An unwavering capacity for equanimity emerges as we are able to be with the movement of neural platforms and gunas and change our relationship to the agitation, clarity, and inertia that life brings.

As discussed in Chapter 3, the Bhagavad Gita's teachings are significant to the yogic perspective of resilience:

> As the mountainous depths of the ocean are unmoved when waters rush into it, so the man unmoved when desires enter him attains a peace that eludes the man of many desires.
>
> (2.70)[4]

The ocean does not stop water from entering it or shifts from occurring within its depths; rather, its vast expanse contains the movement of the currents and animals within. As we learn to connect to awareness, we create depths that allow for the movement of the qualities of body, mind, and environment. Peace follows from the capacity to allow the arising and passing of experience and sensation, to allow the movement of the gunas. According to the Bhagavad Gita, this peace cannot be experienced by one who shuts off from life.

Yoga teaches us to accept and embrace all of life, to not fear what life brings. We need not "flee from the world,"[5] but can instead learn to allow it to come in and teach us. The world then does not "flee from us," as we are able to be more present and nonjudgmental, learning from each experience. Yoga helps us to experience life from a perspective of exploration as we examine our reactions and relationships to body, mind, and environmental stimuli. We begin to notice the natural arising and passing of fear, anger, sadness, and grief without judgment or the creation of tension. We explore those patterns that may perpetuate suffering and inquire into the right actions to enable greater well-being.

A Yoga Therapy Framework for Regulation and Resilience

Yoga therapy looks to affect the underlying gunas and neural platforms, as well as the person's relationship to them, to enhance regulation, resilience, and systemic BPSS well-being. This focus is central to yoga therapy's capacity to influence connected physiological, emotional, and behavioral states or attributes.

Strengthening one's ability to promote sattva guna and activate the social engagement neural platform builds self-regulatory skills as we learn to access physiological restoration, psychological calm, and prosocial behavioral states. The anchor of sattva and the social engagement neural platform provide a capacity to return to safety and calm amidst stressful or difficult life events.

Resilience can be described in a few different ways. One is the ability to move efficiently between guna states and neural platforms as appropriate to the situation. Through greater discernment and interoceptive skill, we learn to identify states of rajas/tamas or defensive mobilization/immobilization and to quickly return to sattva/the social engagement neural platform. Through yogic practices, we can learn to both identify and move between neural platforms and guna states with greater ease. The term *cyclic meditation* captures an analogous alternation between activation and restoration emphasized by some yoga styles. This kind of practice empowers us to recognize naturally fluctuating states and gain proficiency in returning to calm, safe, homeostatic states.

A second way of describing resilience is as a wider range of circumstances in which we can experience safe mobilization and safe immobilization, or balanced sattva with rajas or tamas. From a strong foundation in sattva or social engagement, we learn to withstand and be present to a wider range of stimuli. Consequently, we can tolerate a greater variety of body-mind-environmental activation.

A third way of understanding resilience arises from the realization of all stimuli of the body-mind-environment as awareness. A resilient person experiences eudaimonic well-being, steadfast joy, and equanimity amidst the natural fluctuations of all stimuli. Figure 8.2 depicts this yogic model of resilience, in which we strengthen sattva and navigate the rising and falling of tamas and rajas. (Chapter 11 focuses on practices to enhance resilience.)

Clinical Relevance

Yogic practices can be used to foster sattva and activate the social engagement system as well as to teach new relationships with rajas/tamas and with other

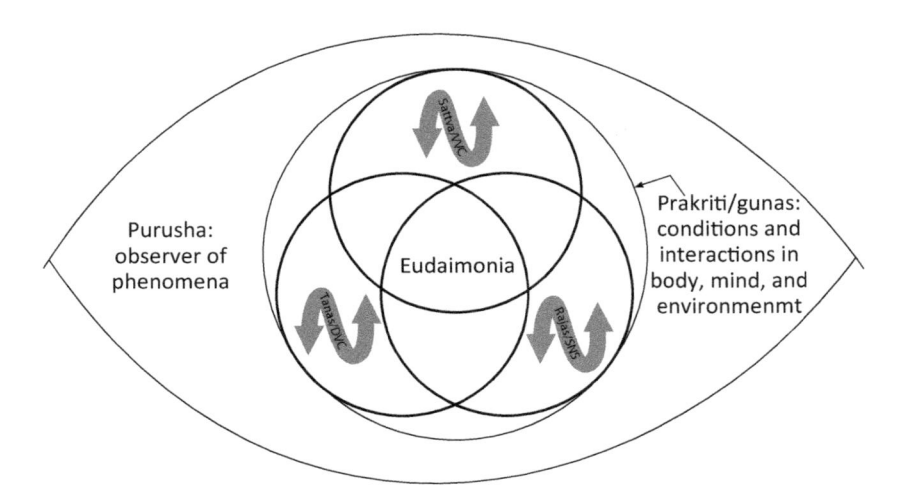

Figure 8.2 Yoga and Polyvagal Theory: Gunas and Neural Platforms.

Notes: In the yogic model of resilience, the outer eye, purusha, observes the natural fluctuations of the body, mind, and environment; the gunas (and neural platforms of polyvagal theory) make up the inner eye, prakriti, which comprises all phenomena. Situated in a state of inner and outer harmony, we realize a sense of contentment, connectedness, and purpose amidst all circumstances and natural fluctuations of the gunas and neural platforms.

VVC = ventral vagal complex; SNS = sympathetic nervous system; DVC = dorsal vagal complex.
Source: Adapted with permission from Sullivan, M. B., Erb, M., Schmalzl, L., Moonaz, S., Noggle Taylor, J., & Porges, S. W. (2018). Yoga therapy and polyvagal theory: The convergence of traditional wisdom and contemporary neuroscience for self-regulation and resilience. *Frontiers in Human Neuroscience, 12,* 67.

neural platforms. Going beyond cultivation of sattva is important, as throughout a lifetime we all continue to encounter stimuli that perpetuate patterns behind suffering. Rather than focusing solely on the light of sattva, we need to create a wider capacity for experiencing the components of safe mobilization, including play, motivation, and activation for healthy and positive change. We can become empowered to be present with pain, tension, agitation, strong emotion, or loss of physical function while maintaining connection to our essential nature, others, and life itself. We learn to experience spiritual and eudaimonic well-being throughout life's circumstances.

In a yoga therapy session, we often start by cultivating the foundation of sattva and parasympathetic activation. This might take the form of restorative postures, soothing movement, calming breathing techniques, or intentions of peace or meaning. From sattva and the activation of the social engagement neural platform, we can work to activate the other gunas and neural platforms and assist clients in an exploration to widen the threshold of tolerance to these other states. For example, we can use movement like a strong bridge or warrior pose to activate the system while simultaneously practicing breathing techniques that activate the parasympathetic nervous system to promote equanimity.

Practical, Specific Application

The practices of yoga work toward the alleviation of suffering and BPSS well-being through integrated top-down neurocognitive and bottom-up neurophysiological processes. I am often asked about "protocols" for yoga therapy to address allopathic conditions, but yoga therapy's effectiveness as a healing practice is not diagnosis-driven. Instead, the practices are meant to be implemented synergistically. Part III of this book explores how selected practices of yoga therapy can be used together to promote regulation of the body and mind (Chapter 9), interoception and discriminative wisdom (Chapter 10), and resilience (Chapter 11). Research supports yoga's capacity to foster compassion and empathy with concurrent effects on autonomic regulation, attention, and affect.[6]

Yoga therapists co-facilitate a self-empowering process through which they adapt practices of philosophy and ethics, postures and movement, breathing techniques, and meditations to meet the needs of the individual. The clinical reasoning process includes assessment along the koshas as well as an understanding of current research, biomedical knowledge, yoga philosophy and its practices, and client needs and values. All of these components are essential to inform the creation and application of the yoga therapy intervention.

Yoga therapists must take medical diagnoses into account for contraindications and other considerations as to what can safely be included in sessions. For example, given a diagnosis of osteoporosis, we would be careful of spinal flexion due to the possible risk of vertebral fracture and might prioritize weight-bearing postures to promote bone strength. With rheumatoid arthritis, the possible degeneration of joints would inform us to focus on balancing joint mobility and stability while being aware of compressive forces.

Yama and Niyama

Chapter 2 introduced the yamas and niyamas as practices of virtues and ethical qualities that align us with right action to actualize dharma. These principles, a foundational element of yoga therapy, help clients to explore their values and needs for greater connection (intrapersonal ⟶ interpersonal ⟶ existential), meaning, and a purpose-filled life to alleviate suffering and promote BPSS well-being.

The Yoga Sutras of Patanjali introduce 10 yamas and niyamas; other texts, such as the Bhagavad Gita, contain more than 30 examples.[7] Examples from the Yoga Sutras and Bhagavad Gita include nonharming, truthfulness, non-stealing, nongrasping, contentment, right effort or self-discipline, self-study, surrender to the divine or to awareness within, compassion, and forgiveness.

Research supports the inclusion of spiritual and ethical components, compared to practicing yoga as an exclusively physical exercise, for improved hedonic and eudaimonic well-being as well as greater physical and mental health benefits including decreased depression and anxiety symptoms and improved mindfulness and cortisol levels.[8]

Experts also support the inclusion of philosophical and ethical principles for clinical populations.[9] Yoga is often perceived as both a way to help a health condition and a spiritual activity,[10] but its spiritual benefits have been reported to become a primary reason for continued practice.[11] This shift to spiritual intention as a motivator to practice may be significant for increasing adherence to physical activity in clinical populations. Yoga can become a vehicle for spiritual growth and transformation as well as a physical activity, mental practice, and facilitator of social connection.

Pranayama

Pranayama is the practice of breath regulation or control. *Prana* means life force, vital force, or breath, and *ayama* means to control or prolong.[12] These practices include ways of manipulating the breath to affect the mind and the flow of prana through the body, and ultimately to further practitioners along the path of yoga for the alleviation of suffering. There are many methods of pranayama including specific ways of inhaling, exhaling, holding the breath, and breathing through one or both nostrils.

Descriptions of pranayama and its importance to yoga can be found in early references to the yogic path and throughout texts such as the Upanishads, Hatha Yoga Pradipika, and Yoga Sutras of Patanjali.[13] The Hatha Yoga Pradipika expresses the close relationship between mind and breath: Wherever one goes, the other follows. When the breath is steady the mind is steady—and vice versa—and we can use the breath as a way to promote steadiness in the mind.[14]

The breath is a powerful bridge between physical and mental processes as well as between conscious and unconscious/subconscious reactions. Our respiratory patterns reflect activation of the parasympathetic and sympathetic systems. Because the underlying autonomic state is influenced by both physiological and psychoemotional input, attention to the breath provides insight into our state of mind-body activation or relaxation. Different emotions such as sadness, anger, happiness, and fear have been shown to be related to distinct cardiorespiratory patterns including respiration variability.[15] Paying attention to our own breathing can help us to recognize our subconscious or unconscious patterns of emotions, thoughts, beliefs, and physiological activations. In addition to reflecting the state of the mind and body, the breath is under voluntary control. Both the insight garnered from noticing breath patterns and the capacity to actively manipulate the breath help us to use pranayama as a powerful method for change.

Research supports the effects of pranayama on neurocognitive, autonomic, pulmonary, and metabolic function and for improving symptoms in clinical populations such as those with anxiety, insomnia, post-traumatic stress disorder, depression, schizophrenia, cardiovascular and respiratory issues, diabetes, and cancer.[16] Specific effects of breath practices include regulation of emotion, attention, and cognitive function and decreased negative affect.[17] In one study, although both breath- and movement-focused practices reduced perceived stress and salivary cortisol, only the breath-focused practice improved attentional control.[18]

Pranayama practices have also been found to shift autonomic nervous system state. Activation of parasympathetic states is thought to influence brain pathways involved in emotional regulation, stress reactivity, higher-order cognitive processes such as decision-making, and the release of prosocial hormones such as oxytocin, which increase the potential for feelings of connection and empathy.[19] This combined influence to promote restorative physiological states, positive psychological states, and emotional regulation mirrors attributes of the social engagement neural platform. Activation of the sympathetic nervous system, which we can also accomplish with specific pranayama, can be useful in clinical populations to promote engagement of the neural platform of safe mobilization and the resilience to move between neural platforms.[20]

The purposeful regulation of breath is taught to bring steadiness and tranquility to the body-mind and as preparation for meditation, promoting qualities of sattva guna.[21] In addition, the prana vayus, or forms of prana, are often taught as related to the movement of breath: The inhale relates to prana vayu and the exhale to apana vayu, the pause between respirations concerns samana vayu, breath into the collarbones concerns udana vayu, and the breath's fluidity reflects the health of vyana vayu.

Asana

Modern depictions of yoga often emphasize the practice of *yoga asana,* or postures. Particularly in the West, asana are often used to symbolize yoga. As a result, many believe yoga practice to be synonymous with development of physical skill, flexibility, and strength. Popular, recognizable postures and sequences such as downward-facing dog, warriors, and sun salutations are, however, recent additions to the compendium of yoga.[22]

According to Mallinson and Singleton, the earlier yogic texts use the word *asana* to describe a way of sitting rather than the postures as they are practiced today. Asana was a prerequisite to work with meditation, breath control, and control of the mind. The Yoga Sutras describe asana as a steady and easy, or comfortable, seat.[23]

Practicing a variety of postures besides ways of sitting became predominant in such texts as the Hatha Yoga Pradipika in the 15th century, proliferated through the 1900s, and continues to grow.[24] Over time, asana has moved from primarily a stable base for seated meditation and breath techniques to a methodology of physical fitness and skill. Today, a nearly infinite number of yoga asana are practiced, with whole schools based on particular movements.

Following from this standpoint, asana provides a means of settling the mind and breath for the deeper inquiry of yoga. Any position that brings ease and steadiness to the body-mind is an asana. This book explores asana as a means of regulation to provide this steady base (Chapter 9), support the development of interoceptive skills (Chapter 10), and cultivate resilience (Chapter 11).

Asana offers benefits that range from gross physical to subtle psychoemotional-spiritual effects.

- **Support of bone health.** Through weight-bearing postures, yoga asana promotes bone density and growth. Standing poses, for example, strengthen the structures of the feet, legs, and spine, whereas plank or hands-and-knees poses strengthen the hands, wrists, and arms.
- **Fall prevention.** Standing postures, one-leg balances, and even hands-and-knees yoga asana can help to challenge and therefore strengthen balance and enhance proprioceptive awareness.

- **Cardiovascular health.** Through both dynamic movements that can provide some aerobic benefit as well as postures that promote relaxation, yoga asana can help to decrease blood pressure and support cardiac health.
- **Respiratory and gastrointestinal mobility/motility.** By maintaining or improving range of motion of the torso, yoga asana can promote optimal diaphragmatic excursion for breathing patterns that activate the parasympathetic nervous system. In turn, this parasympathetic response positively affects cardiovascular, digestive, immune, and endocrine functions for restoration. Another result of increased mobility in the abdominal region is enhanced intestinal motility for healthy digestion. Releasing tension in these regions that affect breathing and digestion supports access to relaxed physiological states.
- **Functional movement for daily life.** Yoga asana can be used to promote musculoskeletal balance, which helps to:
    - support optimal range of motion through both dynamic and static movements that enhance muscular, fascial, and joint mobility;
    - enhance joint stability and muscular strength through movements that require muscular engagement;
    - improve neuromotor control through both movement and specific attention to movement, which enhances the body-mind connection through proprioceptive and interoceptive input; and
    - release muscular tension through postures that promote ease and comfort.

  This improved quality of motion supports function, overall confidence, and belief in the body's ability to participate in daily activities.
- **Support of parasympathetic states.** Specific movements such as posterior pelvic tilting have been found to enhance parasympathetic activation by improving measures of vagal predominance.[25]
- **Influence on emotion and mood.** Studies have looked at how certain emotions correlate to particular movements or body positions.[26] Happiness relates to rising, light, expanding, and freely flowing movements; sadness relates to sinking and heavy movements; anger relates to advancing movements; and fear relates to retreating, condensing movements.
- **Support of body-mind connection.** Asana can be used to develop proprioception and interoception for improved body awareness and mind-body connectivity to support both self-regulation and resilience. Enhanced connection to our physiological and psychoemotional states helps us to cultivate insight into the body-mind relationship and promotes experiences essential to regulation (e.g., peace, calm, safety, relaxation).

- **Challenge to beliefs/past experience and creation of safety in movement.** We can use postures to help uncover experiences of strength, acceptance, or compassion; enhance self-esteem, confidence, and surety; or teach safe movement and address kinesiophobia (fear of movement).

Asana provides an accessible and tangible entryway into the workings of the body-mind and the transformative processes of yoga. In many yogic teachings, asana is practiced first to ready the individual for the deeper and more subtle practices. In addition, some lineages teach that as we connect to our own inner wisdom, spontaneous postures may arise to allow for healing and transformation.

Meditation

Although *meditation* includes various styles and techniques, they all involve mentally based practice that is meant to help us observe and regulate attention, emotion, and physiological activation. Techniques include focused attention to outer or inner objects, mental imagery, mantra, affirmations, chanting, compassion or loving-kindness, specific sense-withdrawal practices, open monitoring, and nondual awareness. Research demonstrates both distinct and shared effects of these different types of mediation on physiology, emotion, and behavior.[27]

The Yoga Sutras outline a continuum of meditation starting with disengagement of the senses from the objects of the outer world. This stage, *pratyahara*, describes the practice of turning the senses inward, away from habitual engagement with outer objects, to cultivate inner attention. Pratyahara represents the shift from breath control and movement toward a more inward-focused practice.

According to Patanjali, from pratyahara the stages of meditation progress from brief to continuous flow of focused, one-pointed attention and to complete absorption. *Dharana* is the initiation of concentrated, one-pointed attention to an internal or external focal point. *Dhyana*, the subsequent stage, is where brief moments of concentration become an unwavering, uninterrupted flow of attention on the object of meditation. In *samadhi*, the continuation of this process of meditation, the distinction between subject and object disappears. The realization of oneself as awareness arises, and all concepts of separation dissolve.

Some types of meditation are as follows:

- **Focused attention** involves directing attention to an external object such as a tree, picture, or statue or to an internal object such as the breath or an

area of the body. To build focus on the object of concentration, the individual is instructed to notice and disengage from other stimuli—thoughts, emotion, sounds—that might arise. Whenever the person notices that the mind has wandered, she draws her attention back to the object of the meditation. Mantra can be considered a type of focused attention meditation, as it includes the verbal or silent repetition of a word, phrase, or sentence. Visualizations also may be a form of focused meditation, as they include creating and maintaining a focus on mental imagery.
- **Sense withdrawal, or pratyahara, meditations** involve purposefully drawing the senses away from the outer world and toward attention to inner sensation.
- **Open monitoring** includes techniques that emphasize a nonjudgmental, nonevaluative noticing of body, mind, and environmental content. The person is taught to cultivate a present-centered, moment-to-moment attention as he observes the rising and falling of thoughts, emotions, physical sensations, and environmental stimuli. This type of meditation encourages an open, accepting attitude: Anything may arise without resistance, and nothing is held onto as it subsides.
- **Loving-kindness *(metta)* and compassion meditations** are intended to help the individual connect to herself and others with feelings of love, joy, and kindness. They facilitate prosocial behavior and connection. Often, the practice directs these feelings to oneself, loved ones, strangers, those who provoke stress, and all beings.
- **Nondual awareness practices** promote experiences of unity by dissolving the boundaries between subject and object, the external and internal. These practices include techniques for deep relaxation, such as *yoga nidra,* or yogic sleep.

Many resources explore the benefits of meditation,[28] which include the following:

- Supporting parasympathetic activation and vagal control can decrease allostatic load and support healthy function, including that of the endocrine, digestive, cardiovascular, and immune systems.
- Focused meditations in particular may aid attentional control and regulation as the person learns to manage distraction by continuously bringing awareness back to the object of focus.
- Structural and functional changes in the brain may affect cognition, executive function, and cognitive control; mood and emotional regulation; body awareness, including proprioceptive and interoceptive processes;

memory; and pain processing. Visualization practices may also affect areas of the brain involved in visual processing and perception. Mantra meditations often include a speech component as the object of focus and so may affect areas of the brain involved in the motor control of speech.
- Meditation practices may promote self-regulatory behaviors via the voluntary regulation of thought, behavior, cognitive and attentional regulation and control, and interoceptive processing.
- Meditation may be used to cultivate prosocial behaviors like compassion or empathy and positive psychological and emotional states like joy.
- Meditation practices can be oriented to improve body-mind connection by prompting awareness of patterns of thought, belief, and behavior and their relationship to physiological state. This insight can help to shift maladaptive or unhealthy patterns to those that encourage well-being.
- Meditation may enhance emotional and mental health, by, for example, improving symptoms of anxiety and depression and increasing emotional regulation and interoceptive processing.

Conclusion

The following chapters consider the application of selected practices in yoga therapy: how yama, niyama, asana, pranayama, and meditation can support systemic body-mind regulation (Chapter 9), healthy and adaptive interoception and discriminative wisdom (Chapter 10), and body-mind resilience (Chapter 11).

An essential part of working with others is curiosity, creativity, and exploration—partnering with our clients on a path of discovery. Each person is an amalgam of experience presenting in a certain way at a certain time, a presentation that will be different in the next moment. The theories, research, and practices provided in this book are meant to support the creative process of clinical thinking.

I have found that scientific knowledge and research provide invaluable inspiration for the exploration and application of yoga philosophy and practices. This background helps to explain the practices to clients and healthcare professionals and points toward best practices and potential limitations. Equally, and perhaps more importantly, clients have helped me to challenge my own perceptions, ideas, and biases and to continuously explore the practices in reference to each moment in time. Physical therapist and yoga therapist Matthew Taylor writes about the essentially fluid use of yoga therapy in working with pain in *Yoga Therapy as a Creative Response to Pain*.[29]

As a clinician, I am constantly inspired by the ever-changing application of yogic practices driven by the client's needs. Practicing a healthcare discipline in this way is an art and a science, a process of being attuned to the client, to oneself (including our own clinical expertise), and to the science and philosophy behind the practices.

The examples offered in this book are not meant to be interpreted as the sole methods for this process. These examples, which represent practices I have used in my personal and professional experience, are provided to give specific practical ideas as well as to foster creativity and inspire more ideas. I hope that readers will consider how yoga furthers intentions of regulation, interoception and wisdom, and resilience. These theories and practices can be part of an exploration within the therapeutic relationship to determine what is needed and arising in any particular moment. I invite you to be creative in the ways in which you apply this information and support the process of discovery along the journey toward well-being.

Notes

1. Craig, A. D. (2015). *How do you feel? An interoceptive moment with your neurobiological self.* Princeton, NJ: Princeton University Press; Porges, S. W. (1993). The infant's sixth sense: Awareness and regulation of bodily processes. *Zero to Three: Bulletin of the National Center for Clinical Infant Programs, 14,* 12–16; Farb, N., Daubenmier, J., Price, C. J., Gard, T., Kerr, C., Dunn, B. D., … Mehling, W. E. (2015). Interoception, contemplative practice and health. *Frontiers in Psychology, 6,* 763. doi:10.3389/fpsyg.2015.00763; Strigo, I. A., & Craig, A. D. (2016). Interoception, homeostatic emotions and sympathovagal balance. *Philosophical Transactions of the Royal Society B: Biological Sciences, 371,* 20160010. doi:10.1098/rstb.2016.0010
2. Craig, *How do you feel?*; Strigo & Craig, Interoception, homeostatic emotions and sympathovagal balance; Farb et al., Interoception, contemplative practice and health; Porges, S. W. (2011). threats and safety. *Zero to Three, 24*(5), 19–24; Porges, S. W. (2011). *The polyvagal theory: Neurophysiological foundations of emotions, attachment, communication, and self-regulation* (1st ed.). New York: W. W. Norton; Ceunen, E., Vlaeyen, J. W., & Van Diest, I. (2016). On the Origin of Interoception. *Frontiers in Psychology, 7,* 743. doi:10.3389/fpsyg.2016. 00743; Haase, L., Stewart, J. L., Youssef, B., May, A. C., Isakovic, S., Simmons, A. N., … Paulus, M. (2016). When the brain does not adequately feel the body: Links between low resilience and interoception. *Biological Psychology, 113,* 37–45. doi:10.1016/j.biopsycho. 2015.11.004
3. Sullivan, M. B., Erb, M., Schmalzl, L., Moonaz, S., Noggle Taylor, J., & Porges, S. W. (2018). Yoga therapy and polyvagal theory: The convergence of traditional wisdom and contemporary neuroscience for self-regulation and resilience. *Frontiers in Human Neuroscience, 12,* 67.
4. Miller, B. S. (Trans.) (1986). *The Bhagavad-Gita: Krishna's counsel in time of war.* New York: Bantam Classics.

5. Miller, *The Bhagavad-Gita*, 12.15 (p. 113).
6. Fiori, F., Aglioti, S. M., & David, N. (2017). Interactions between body and social awareness in yoga. *Journal of Alternative and Complementary Medicine, 23*(3), 227–233; Mackenzie, M. J., Carlson, L. E., Paskevich, D. M., Ekkekakis, P., Wurz, A. J., Wytsma, K., … & Culos-Reed, S. N. (2014). Associations between attention, affect and cardiac activity in a single yoga session for female cancer survivors: An enactive neurophenomenology-based approach. *Consciousness and Cognition, 27*, 129–146.
7. Gupta, B. (2006). Bhagavad Gītā as duty and virtue ethics: Some reflections. *Journal of Religious Ethics, 34*(3), 373–395.
8. Gaiswinkler, L., & Unterrainer, H. F. (2016). The relationship between yoga involvement, mindfulness and psychological well-being. *Complementary Therapies in Medicine, 26*, 123–127; Ivtzan, I., & Jegatheeswaran, S. (2015). The yoga boom in western society: Practitioners' spiritual vs. physical intentions and their impact on psychological wellbeing. *Journal of Yoga & Physical Therapy, 5*(204), 2; Ivtzan, I., & Papantoniou, A. (2014). Yoga meets positive psychology: Examining the integration of hedonic (gratitude) and eudaimonic (meaning) wellbeing in relation to the extent of yoga practice. *Journal of Bodywork and Movement Therapies, 18*(2), 183–189; Smith, J. A., Greer, T., Sheets, T., & Watson, S. (2011). Is there more to yoga than exercise? *Alternative Therapies in Health & Medicine, 17*(3), 22–29;
9. de Manincor, M., Bensoussan, A., Smith, C., Fahey, P., & Bourchier, S. (2015). Establishing key components of yoga interventions for reducing depression and anxiety, and improving well-being: A Delphi method study. *BMC Complementary and Alternative Medicine, 15*(1), 85.
10. Quilty, M. T., Saper, R. B., Goldstein, R., & Khalsa, S. B. S. (2013). Yoga in the real world: Perceptions, motivators, barriers, and patterns of use. *Global Advances in Health and Medicine, 2*(1), 44–49.
11. Ivtzan & Jegatheeswaran, The yoga boom in western society; Park, C. L., Riley, K. E., Bedesin, E., & Stewart, V. M. (2016). Why practice yoga? Practitioners' motivations for adopting and maintaining yoga practice. *Journal of Health Psychology, 21*(6), 887–896.
12. Mallinson, J., & Singleton, M. (2017). *Roots of yoga*. London: Penguin; Telles, S., & Naveen, K. V. (2008). Voluntary breath regulation in yoga: Its relevance and physiological effects. *Biofeedback, 36*(2), 70–73.
13. Mallinson & Singleton, *Roots of yoga*; Telles & Naveen, Voluntary breath regulation in yoga.
14. Saraswati, M., Saraswati, S., & Svātmārāma. (2012). *Hatha yoga pradipika = Light on hatha yoga: Including the original Sanskrit text of the Hatha yoga pradipika with translation in English*, p. 642. Munger, India: Yoga Publications Trust; Telles & Naveen, Voluntary breath regulation in yoga.
15. Rainville, P., Bechara, A., Naqvi, N., & Damasio, A. R. (2006). Basic emotions are associated with distinct patterns of cardiorespiratory activity. *International Journal of Psychophysiology, 61*(1), 5–18.
16. Brown, R. P., Gerbarg, P. L., & Muench, F. (2013). Breathing practices for treatment of psychiatric and stress-related medical conditions. *Psychiatric Clinics, 36*(1), 121–140; Telles, S., Singh, N., & Puthige, R. (2013). Changes in P300 following alternate nostril yoga breathing and breath awareness. *BioPsychoSocial Medicine, 7*(1), 11; Mason, H., Vandoni, M., Debarbieri, G., Codrons, E., Ugargol, V., & Bernardi, L. (2013). Cardiovascular and respiratory effect of yogic slow breathing in the yoga beginner:

What is the best approach? *Evidence-Based Complementary and Alternative Medicine, 2013*, 743504; Saoji, A. A., Raghavendra, B. R., & Manjunath, N. K. (2018). Effects of yogic breath regulation: A narrative review of scientific evidence. *Journal of Ayurveda and Integrative Medicine, 10*(1). doi:10.1016/j.jaim.2017.07.008
17. Brown, Gerbarg, & Muench, Breathing practices for treatment of psychiatric and stress-related medical conditions.
18. Schmalzl, L., Powers, C., Zanesco, A. P., Yetz, N., Groessl, E. J., & Saron, C. D. (2018). The effect of movement-focused and breath-focused yoga practice on stress parameters and sustained attention: A randomized controlled pilot study. *Consciousness and Cognition, 65*, 109–125.
19. Brown, R. P., & Gerbarg, P. L. (2005). Sudarshan kriya yogic breathing in the treatment of stress, anxiety, and depression: Part I—Neurophysiologic model. *Journal of Alternative and Complementary Medicine, 11*(1), 189–201. https://doi.org/10.1089/acm.2005.11.189; Brown, Gerbarg, & Muench, Breathing practices for treatment of psychiatric and stress-related medical conditions; Mason et al., Cardiovascular and respiratory effect of yogic slow breathing in the yoga beginner; Sinha, A. N. (2013). Assessment of the effects of pranayama/alternate nostril breathing on the parasympathetic nervous system in young adults. *Journal of Clinical and Diagnostic Research, 7*(5), 821–823. doi:10.7860/JCDR/2013/4750.2948; Telles, Singh, & Puthige, Changes in P300 following alternate nostril yoga breathing and breath awareness; Brown, Gerbarg, & Muench, Breathing practices for treatment of psychiatric and stress-related medical conditions.
20. Bhavanani, A. B., Ramanathan, M., & Madanmohan. (2015). Single session of integrated "silver yoga" program improves cardiovascular parameters in senior citizens. *Journal of Intercultural Ethnopharmacology, 4*(2), 134–137; Raghuraj, P., & Telles, S. (2008). Immediate effect of specific nostril manipulating yoga breathing practices on autonomic and respiratory variables. *Applied Psychophysiology and Biofeedback, 33*(2), 65–75; Telles & Naveen, Voluntary breath regulation in yoga; Telles, S., Singh, N., & Balkrishna, A. (2011). Heart rate variability changes during high frequency yoga breathing and breath awareness. *BioPsychoSocial Medicine, 5*(1), 4.
21. Miller, B. S. (1996). *Yoga: Discipline of freedom: The yoga sutra attributed to Patanjali.* Berkeley, CA: University of California Press; Muktibodhananda, *Hatha yoga pradipika.*
22. Singleton, M. (2010). *Yoga body: The origins of modern posture practice.* New York, NY: Oxford University Press.
23. Miller, *Yoga: Discipline of freedom.*
24. Mallinson & Singleton, *Roots of yoga.*
25. Cottingham, J. T., Porges, S. W., & Lyon, T. (1988). Effects of soft tissue mobilization (rolfing pelvic lift) on parasympathetic tone in two age groups. *Journal of the American Physical Therapy Association, 68*(3), 352–356; Cottingham, J. T., Porges, S. W., & Richmond, K. (1988). Shifts in pelvic inclination angle and parasympathetic tone produced by rolfing soft tissue manipulation. *Journal of the American Physical Therapy Association, 68*(9), 1364–1370.
26. Shafir, T., Tsachor, R. P., & Welch, K. B. (2016). Emotion regulation through movement: Unique sets of movement characteristics are associated with and enhance basic emotions. *Frontiers in Psychology, 6.* https://doi.org/10.3389/fpsyg.2015.02030; Tsachor, R. P., & Shafir, T. (2017). A somatic movement approach to fostering emotional resiliency through Laban movement analysis. *Frontiers in Human Neuroscience, 11.* https://doi.org/10.3389/fnhum.2017.00410

27. Fox, K. C. R., Dixon, M. L., Nijeboer, S., Girn, M., Floman, J. L., Lifshitz, M., ... Christoff, K. (2016). Functional neuroanatomy of meditation: A review and meta-analysis of 78 functional neuroimaging investigations. *Neuroscience & Biobehavioral Reviews, 65*, 208–228.

28. Fox et al., Functional neuroanatomy of meditation; Fox, K. C. R., Nijeboer, S., Dixon, M. L., Floman, J. L., Ellamil, M., Rumak, S. P., ... Christoff, K. (2014). Is meditation associated with altered brain structure? A systematic review and meta-analysis of morphometric neuroimaging in meditation practitioners. *Neuroscience & Biobehavioral Reviews, 43*, 48–73; Fredrickson, B. L., Cohn, M. A., Coffey, K. A., Pek, J., & Finkel, S. M. (2008). Open hearts build lives: Positive emotions, induced through loving-kindness meditation, build consequential personal resources. *Journal of Personality and Social Psychology, 95*(5), 1045–1062; Galvin, J. A., Benson, H., Deckro, G. R., Fricchione, G. L., & Dusek, J. A. (2006). The relaxation response: Reducing stress and improving cognition in healthy aging adults. *Complementary Therapies in Clinical Practice, 12*(3), 186–191; Goyal, M., Singh, S., Sibinga, E. M. S., Gould, N. F., Rowland-Seymour, A., Sharma, R., ... Haythornthwaite, J. A. (2014). Meditation programs for psychological stress and well-being: A systematic review and meta-analysis. *JAMA Internal Medicine, 174*(3), 357–368; Hasenkamp, W., Wilson-Mendenhall, C. D., Duncan, E., & Barsalou, L. W. (2012). Mind wandering and attention during focused meditation: A fine-grained temporal analysis of fluctuating cognitive states. *NeuroImage, 59*(1), 750–760; Tang, Y.-Y., Hölzel, B. K., & Posner, M. I. (2015). The neuroscience of mindfulness meditation. *Nature Reviews: Neuroscience, 16*(4), 213–225; Zeng, X., Chiu, C. P. K., Wang, R., Oei, T. P. S., & Leung, F. Y. K. (2015). The effect of loving-kindness meditation on positive emotions: A meta-analytic review. *Frontiers in Psychology, 6*. https://doi.org/10.3389/fpsyg.2015.01693

29. Taylor, M. J. (2018). *Yoga therapy as a creative response to pain*. London: Singing Dragon.

PART III

Applied Philosophy and Science for Health and Well-Being

Setting the Stage for Well-Being

9

Practices for Cultivating Sattva Guna and Regulating the Body-Mind

This chapter provides specific examples and ideas for practicing yama/niyama, asana, pranayama, and meditation to foster sattva guna and systemic body-mind regulation. This is not an exhaustive list of possible yogic practices; from a neurophysiological perspective, however, these practices are among those that activate the social engagement neural platform, leading to relaxed physiological, positive psychological, and prosocial behavioral states. From a social and spiritual perspective, they foster a sense of connection (intrapersonal ⟶ interpersonal ⟶ existential), meaning-making, and purpose.

Yama and Niyama

As foundational practices of ethical inquiry, yama and niyama can be used to examine and shift patterns of physiological, psychological, and behavioral activation to cultivate the attributes of sattva guna and the social engagement neural platform. These practices help us to recognize how our personal values both shape the experience of suffering and provide a path for easing it. Living in alignment with one's values empowers discovery of greater personal and interpersonal connections and underpins a purposeful life.

Often, people cite Patanjali's yamas and niyamas as the ethical practices of yoga. However, other texts such as the Mahabharata and its Bhagavad Gita include many other ethical principles relevant to the yoga therapeutic process.[1] I find it most useful to discuss with clients what kinds of values-based questions might be arising for them around current struggles. Based on such conversations, we can work with any ethical principle to form intentional practices relevant to their circumstances.

Aristotle taught the *golden mean* as a method of reflection on ethical qualities, which he considered guideposts to eudaimonia. The individual is instructed to explore the excess, deficiency, and middle ground for any ethical quality, such as humility or generosity. Next, she assesses her tendencies along this continuum to consider how to move toward the mean of the ethical quality (Figure 9.1). This practice of the golden mean is a powerful method of inquiry into one's values.

The Golden Mean in Practice: Example Qualities to Explore

Humility

A deficiency of humility would be seen, for example, in arrogance, conceit, self-importance, or a sense of superiority. Excess humility is represented by a lack of self-respect, self-esteem, or self-worth; people with too much humility may be overly insecure or even exhibit self-hatred.

Generosity

A deficiency in generosity might be seen in stinginess or unwillingness to give to others either emotionally or physically. Giving so much of oneself that one does not engage in self-care or healthy boundaries may represent excess generosity.

Courage

A deficiency of courage could be experienced as excessive worry about non-dangerous stimuli or a fear of change. Reckless action that may harm oneself or others is an example of excess courage.

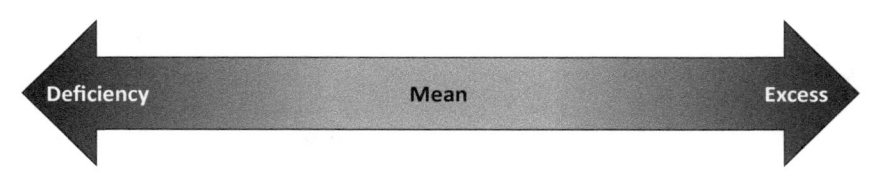

Figure 9.1 Aristotle's Golden Mean Can Be Used to Inquire Into Ethical Qualities Including the Yogic Yamas and Niyamas.

Patience

Deficient patience might be represented by impulsiveness that results in jumping to conclusions, acting based on habitual tendencies, or being unwilling to allow sufficient time for processes of change. Excess patience would be, for example, reluctance to take action even when called for.

Ahimsa: Nonharming

We can also consider the commonly cited yamas and niyamas through the lens of the golden mean. Deficiency in the yama of ahimsa might be seen when people cause harm to themselves or others, including negative self-beliefs and negative self-talk, as well as harmful emotional states or actions. Excess ahimsa would be represented by a person living in such fear of hurting others that they fail to meet their own needs and are unable to take care of themselves. Remaining in a harmful situation is one example.

Satya: Truthfulness

Insufficient satya would be seen in difficulty with speaking and living in a truthful, authentic manner. Deficient satya could also include not being honest about one's own needs or avoiding actions that would benefit oneself or others. Excess satya might include projecting your beliefs onto others in an inconsiderate, thoughtless, or insensitive way. Stating opinion—your truth—as fact or the only possibility, or misunderstanding that your truth is not someone else's truth, also represents excess satya. Telling the truth at the expense of nonharming is likewise excess satya.

Santosha: Contentment

Deficient santosha would be seen in an inability to find serenity or ease—in other words, being discontented. The feeling of never having enough or things never being what you think they should be is a deficiency of santosha. An excess might show up as unwillingness or lack of motivation to change or to explore new ideas or experiences.

Any yama or niyama can be examined on the continuum of the golden mean in this way. Practice 9.2 offers examples of other yamas and niyamas.

> **Practice 9.1 A Yogic Practice of the Golden Mean**
>
> Gather writing materials and find a comfortable seat.
> This practice focuses on exploring values important to you. How do you define their excess, deficiency, and middle way, and where do your tendencies fall on the continuum? What does it mean to find and live in the golden mean of these values?
>
> - Examples of the virtues or values you might want to work with include humility, courage, patience, forgiveness, compassion, acceptance, nonharming, contentment, kindness, and truth.
> - Choose a value and write a few words or sentences about its excess and deficiency in your life.
> - Write down how you conceive of this value's golden mean and where you fall on this continuum.
>
> Sit or lie down comfortably and close your eyes or soften your gaze. In your meditative posture, explore the following questions:
>
> - Is there an image, word, or affirmation that strengthens the idea of the golden mean of this value? Is there a memory that helps you to access this middle path?
> - Can you bring into your body a feeling of aligning with the golden mean of this value? Where would it be? What does it feel like (e.g., open, grounded, energetic, expansive, strong)? Is there a posture or movement that you could create to strengthen the feeling in your body?
> - Imagine a situation in your life that you could bring this experience to. How does the image, word, or physical sensation help you to remember this virtue? Might you use this as a daily practice to strengthen your alignment with this virtue in action, thought, and emotional state?

Additional Practices of Yama and Niyama

See Chapter 2 for a practice (Practice 2.1, p. 33) that focuses on the virtues in relation to dharma.

Yoga therapist Tina Paul has created an insightful list of reflective questions and ideas to prompt discussion or journaling, or as a foundation for meditations on the yamas and niyamas (see Practice 9.2).

Practice 9.2 Reflection on Yama and Niyama: Possible Practical Applications

	Application
Yama (personal discipline)	
Ahimsa (nonharming)	• Observe your thoughts, feelings, and actions and notice patterns of judgment, criticism, anger, or irritation toward yourself and others. • Practice nonharming with your body, mind/emotions, and behavior/interactions with others.
Satya (truthfulness)	• Notice thoughts, feelings, words, and behavior and how to meet each moment from truth. • Notice interactions with others and how to meet each with truth and kindness.
Asteya (nonstealing)	• Be mindful of stealing time, energy, or the spotlight from others or yourself. • Does a constant rush to achieve steal from your present moment?
Brahmacharya (conservation of energy; walking with Brahman)	• Practice moderation in activities. • Practice control over physical impulses, emotions, and thoughts. • Notice when your thoughts and actions align with your most authentic and essential nature and when they veer away.
Aparigraha (nongrasping)	• Practice contentment and gratitude for yourself, others, and your life. • Notice when you are focused on the next thing or looking for contentment outside yourself.
Niyama (observance)	
Saucha (purity, cleanliness)	• Notice the thoughts, beliefs, and behaviors that lead you away from or closer to your authentic, essential nature.
Santosha (contentment)	• Notice when you are focused on the next thing or looking for contentment outside yourself. • Notice the energy you expend toward others and on outer activities/achievements. • Write a gratitude journal.

continued

> **Practice 9.2 continued**
>
> | | Application |
> |---|---|
> | *Niyama (observance)* | |
> | Tapas (heat, self-discipline) | • Notice persistence and determination in your practice of yoga and in pursuing your goals and intentions; notice any rigidity or lack of persistence. |
> | Svadhyaya (self-study) | • Study wisdom teachings.
• Develop a sense of curiosity about yourself—your beliefs, thoughts, emotions, behaviors, and interactions with others and life.
• Practice connecting to nonjudgmental witnessing and noticing of body, mind, and environment. |
> | Ishvara pranidhana (surrender) | • Notice unhealthy attachments or beliefs that may create suffering or pain.
• What does it mean to let go, surrender, or allow life to flow?
• Practice present-moment appreciation and gratitude as well as nonjudgmental noticing of what is. |
>
> *Source:* Adapted from T. Paul, personal communication, May 1, 2017.

Asana

Patanjali's definition of *asana* supports an intention of promoting relaxed body-mind states and sattva guna. Any body position that includes a relaxation of effort—and is steady and comfortable—can be an asana. Asana need not be limited to the movements typically thought of as yoga postures. Some people may use activities like running, swimming, or dancing in the same intentional ways.

In yoga therapy, we can work with clients to explore positions or exercises that support ease and steadiness in the body and calm and contentment of the mind, which in turn support attributes of compassion and loving-kindness.

Postures for Regulation

A common misconception is that restorative postures or forward folds are always relaxing and the best choice to facilitate the calm and ease needed to support body-mind regulation. For some, however, the abdominal compression or restricted respiration in a seated forward bend or child's pose may be agitating. Remaining in restorative postures for long holds, even when supported, can trigger discomfort, anxiety, or pain. I often find this with people who have more mobility in their joints or less stability in their bodies and in those who may be fearful or have difficulty with stillness. In these cases, the long holds of so-called restorative practices can increase stress, strain, or discomfort.

In other words, a practice that is regulating and restorative to one person may be activating and agitating to another. Similarly, I have heard the claim that backbends are activating or even anxiety-provoking. However, for some, the openness of the area around the heart and easy breath created in a backbend fosters positive, relaxed states of the body-mind, with sattvic qualities (peacefulness, lucidity, buoyancy, connectedness). Depending on the yoga therapist's intention and cueing and on the client's individual history, nearly any posture can have an effect spanning from the facilitation of calm, open, positive states to agitation, fear, and vulnerability.

In working with asana to cultivate systemic regulation, the language and perspective of curiosity, inquiry, and discovery are essential. As we give ideas around movement and postures that may be beneficial for encouraging sattva guna, notice when rigidity about "right" and "wrong" comes into play and instead remember to look to what is arising for the person in the moment. The art of yoga therapy requires us to create a dialogue with clients to investigate whether they are experiencing the qualities of sattva guna and the social engagement neural platform. We can both observe the client and ask them whether a posture is facilitating safety, relaxation, equanimity, or contentment or having the opposite effect.

Theoretical Perspectives

Although the particular asana that support sattva guna, the social engagement neural platform, and relaxed body-mind states are unique to the individual, a few general principles can guide our exploration with clients.

190 Applied Philosophy and Science

- We can support activation of the parasympathetic nervous system through body position, relaxation of muscle tension, and optimization of respiratory function.
    - **Postures that the individual perceives as safe and comfortable and encourage muscular relaxation.** Examples include constructive rest, supported bridge, supine rest with neck support, legs up the wall, supine bound angle, and mountain brook (see Figures 9.2, 9.3, 9.6, 9.9, 9.12, and 9.13).
    - **Postures that help to create mobility in the trunk for greater diaphragmatic excursion optimize respiratory function and parasympathetic activation** (as discussed in Chapter 8). Such positions could include any static or dynamic, active or passive sidebends, backbends, twists, or forward bends.
    - **Positions such as posterior pelvic tilting have been shown to help with PNS activation.**[2] Examples include child's pose, supine knees to chest, and cat stretch.
- We can support positive, relaxed emotional states and prosocial behaviors through particular positions and enhance body-mind connection through the development of healthy interoceptive skills and improved body awareness.
    - As mentioned in Chapter 8, emotional states of happiness are related to rising, light, expanding, free-flowing movements.[3] We can use passive or active, static or dynamic backbends, standing postures, or rhythmic movements to explore how particular actions support positive emotional states. Examples include supported bridge, supported bound angle, mountain brook, and supported fish.
    - As described in Chapters 7 and 8, healthy interoception and body awareness are also related to self-regulation and prosocial behaviors.[4] Chapter 10 outlines more in-depth inquiry for the development of these skills, but we can start this process with simple inquiry in any posture or movement. For example, a body scan in any position facilitates noticing different parts of the body, how they are moving, or where they are in space. Bringing attention to habitual ways of holding tension in different areas and mindfully engaging certain muscle groups during asana are additional possibilities.
- We can support the emergence of sattvic qualities like clarity, luminosity, and buoyancy through the above two principles. In addition, we can use postures that help shift unbalanced rajas or tamas to sattva. For example, activating postures that require muscular engagement, such as tree or warriors, could shift unbalanced tamas to sattva. We could also use

restorative and still postures or gentle, rhythmic movement to bring unbalanced rajas to sattva.
- We can support greater musculoskeletal balance, neuromotor control, and enhanced proprioceptive awareness to help people access greater physical ease, stability, surety, and so on. These concepts, which both optimize function and improve body awareness, are detailed below.

Understanding Musculoskeletal Balance for Body-Mind Regulation

In my opinion, achieving musculoskeletal balance means helping clients to develop the optimal range of motion, strength, stability, and ease needed for their life activities, as well as the capacity to release muscular tension when at rest.

One of the biggest influences in my work with clients has been Vladimir Janda's neuromuscular approach. His focus on the interdependence between the muscular and nervous systems blends well with the information I have learned through yoga and clinical experience. Janda describes characteristic patterns of muscular "tightness" and "weakness" (described briefly below and in Definitions: Terminology for Understanding Musculoskeletal Imbalance, p. 192) that arise from pain, pathology, or any kind of physical dysfunction. These patterns of imbalances have a cyclical effect as they perpetuate dysfunctional movement, which can also contribute to experiences of pain and, in turn, to greater imbalance. We can learn to look for these functional muscular patterns of tightness, shortness, or weakness[5] and to help relax, mobilize, and strengthen these muscles, respectively. Understanding common patterns of imbalance, in addition to assessment by a trained professional, can help identify asana to increase range and ease of motion; relax held tensions; improve body awareness through proprioceptive and interoceptive cueing; and mindfully engage muscles for greater stability, strength, and support in movement.

Length, tone, and strength are independent of one another and can be found in any combination. For example, the pelvic floor muscles are often found to be both tight (have increased tone) and weak, the quadriceps both short and weak, and the iliopsoas both tight and weak with or without normal length. Recognizing this complexity is important, as clients bring with them subjective experiences, noting, for instance, that an area feels "tight," "stuck," or "weak." These experiences could be due to increased or decreased tension or tone, shortness, even weakness—or any combination thereof. The area could lack mobility and working to increase range of motion may help; the area could also be guarding

> **Definitions: Terminology for Understanding Musculoskeletal Imbalance**
>
> **Muscle length:** optimal muscle length allows for ease of range of motion of a joint for functional activity. For example, shortened pectoralis muscles may round the shoulders forward and limit full shoulder flexion (the ability to raise the arms overhead).
>
> **Muscle tone:** amount of contraction or engagement a muscle has in its resting state, demonstrated by the amount of resistance the muscle has to being lengthened when it is at rest. High tone means that the muscle holds a higher amount of tension at rest and more strongly resists lengthening; low tone means the muscle is more easily lengthened passively. When a muscle has high tone, it often subjectively feels tight.
>
> **Muscle strength:** ability of a muscle to contract against a force. Is the body able to meet the individual's needs, such as climbing stairs or lifting? Increasing the stability of the body is a form of strengthening focused on helping to maintain joint alignment, congruence, and ease of motion.
>
> **Muscular weakness/inhibition:** when muscles are not engaging adequately or appropriately to meet the demand put upon them, they are said to be weak. *Muscular inhibition* refers to weakness in which the muscle does not engage as it normally would to meet demand. Muscles often become inhibited as a result of injury or pain (e.g., quadriceps after knee surgery or transverse abdominals in low back dysfunction). Mindful, conscious engagement of these muscles with movement must then be relearned.

or have increased tension and relaxation may help. Still another alternative is underlying instability and weakness contributing to increased tension and the feeling of tightness. "Stretching" the tightness may actually perpetuate the instability and tension with a guarding response, making the experience of discomfort worse; however, stabilizing and strengthening the area may release tension and alleviate discomfort.

Determining these musculoskeletal imbalances for specific applications relies on skilled assessment. However, there are common imbalances—places that tend to have increased or decreased tone, loss of mobility, or insufficient stability or strength—that both result from and contribute to discomfort or injury (see Table 9.1). Understanding and working with these patterns can

Setting the Stage for Well-Being 193

Table 9.1 Common Patterns of Muscular Imbalance

Area of Dysfunction	Weak or Inhibited Muscles	Tight and/or Short Muscles
Low back, hip, knee	Transverse abdominals Gluteus medius/minimus Gluteus maximus Pelvic floor Quadriceps	Iliopsoas Hamstrings Adductors Pelvic floor Quadriceps Piriformis
Shoulder, neck	Lower and middle trapezius Serratus anterior Deep cervical flexors	Upper trapezius Levator scapulae Pectoralis major and minor Latissimus dorsi

help to create a balance of physical relaxation, mobility, and stability for the promotion of sattva guna, regulation of the body-mind, and activation of the social engagement neural platform. The sections below illustrate some of my favorite examples for these intentions.

Postures to Release Commonly Tight Areas

These include supportive positions that encourage the relaxation of effort and help to release tension in the soft tissues such as muscles and fascia. Examples are shown in Figures 9.2 to 9.6.

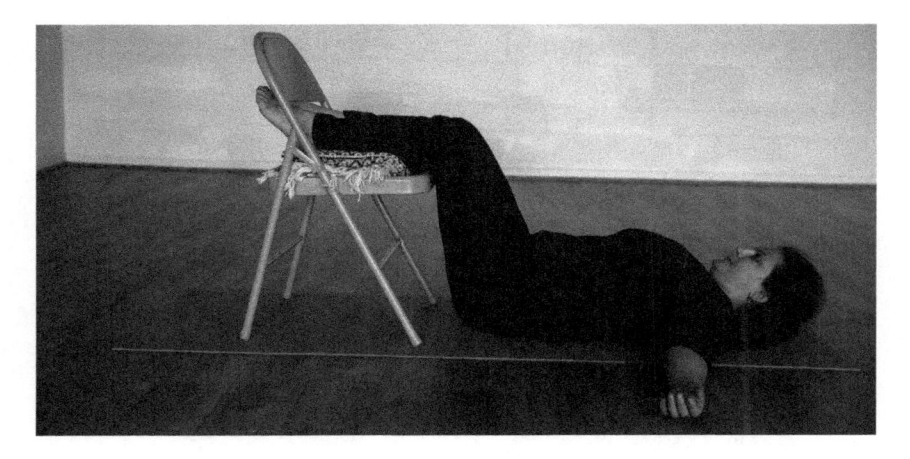

Figure 9.2 Constructive Rest.

Note: Releases the hip flexors (iliopsoas, rectus femoris, tensor fascia latae [TFL], etc.), hamstrings, pelvis, low back. Lie supine with legs supported at 90 degrees of hip and knee flexion.

194 Applied Philosophy and Science

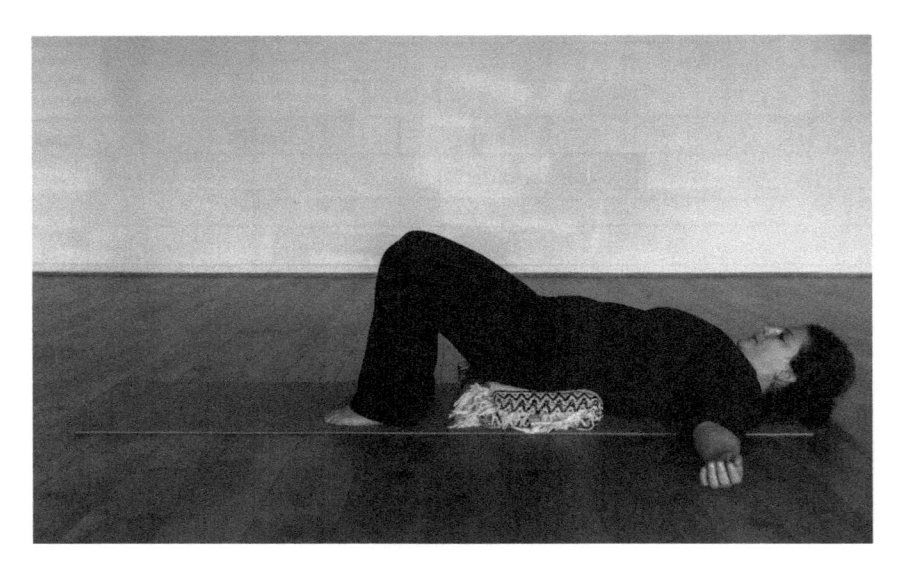

Figure 9.3 Supported Bridge.

Note: Releases the muscles around the pelvis including the pelvic floor. Lie supine with two or more blankets under the pelvis.

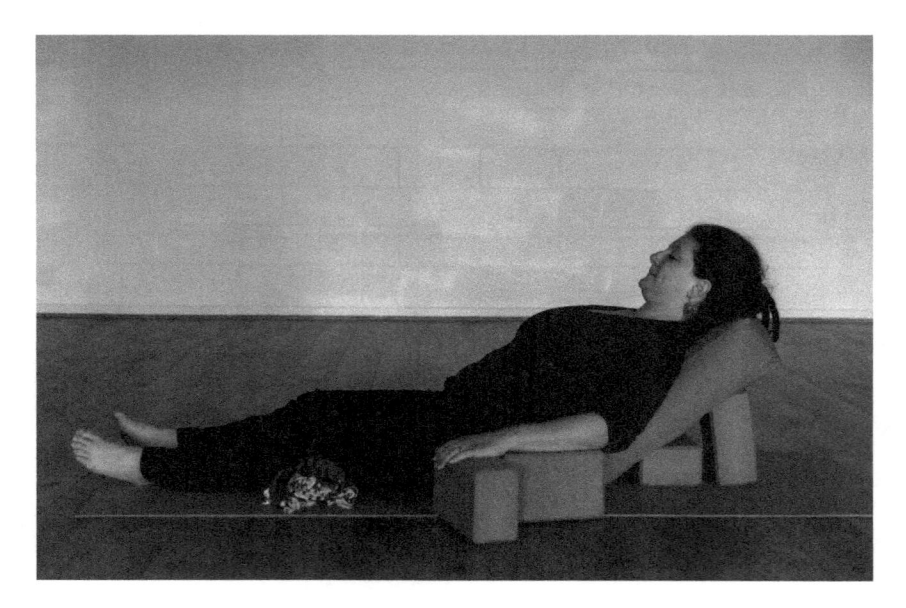

Figure 9.4 Supported Incline Rest.

Note: Supports the body in an inclined posture to facilitate relaxation.

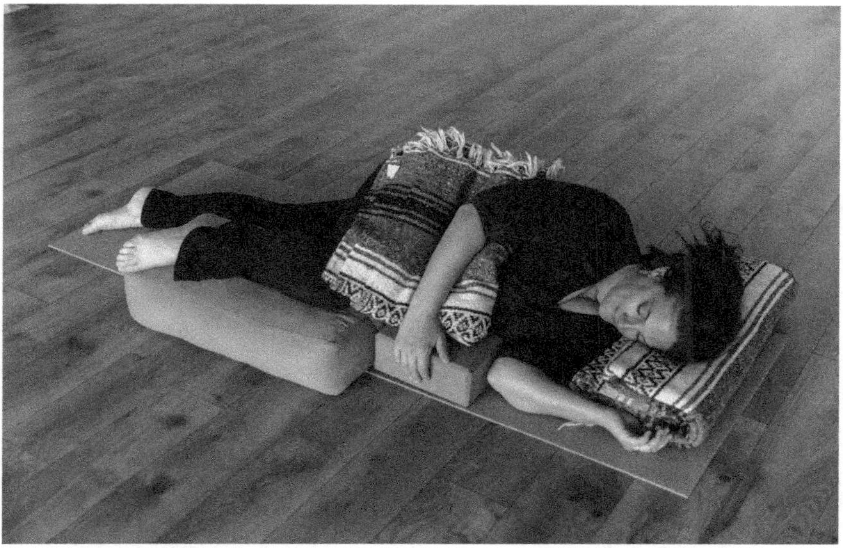

Setting the Stage for Well-Being 195

Figure 9.5 Supported Sidelying.
Note: Alternative support to comfortably facilitate relaxation.

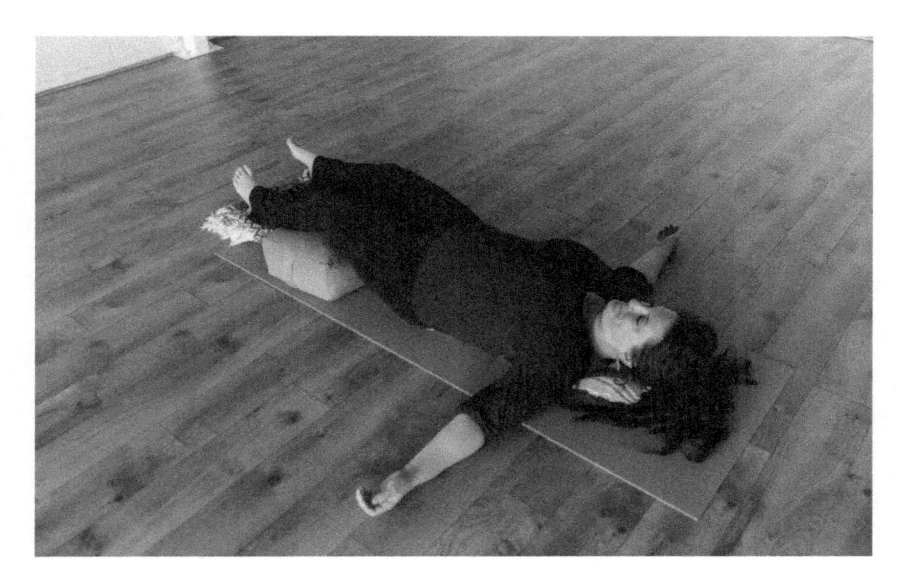

Figure 9.6 Starfish.
Note: Facilitates supported relaxation with mild chest opening. Roll a blanket vertically under the spine from sacrum to head.

Postures to Mobilize and Lengthen Commonly Short Muscles and Fascia

These can be done with careful consideration to proprioceptive input and supporting joint stability, as shown in Figures 9.7 to 9.15.

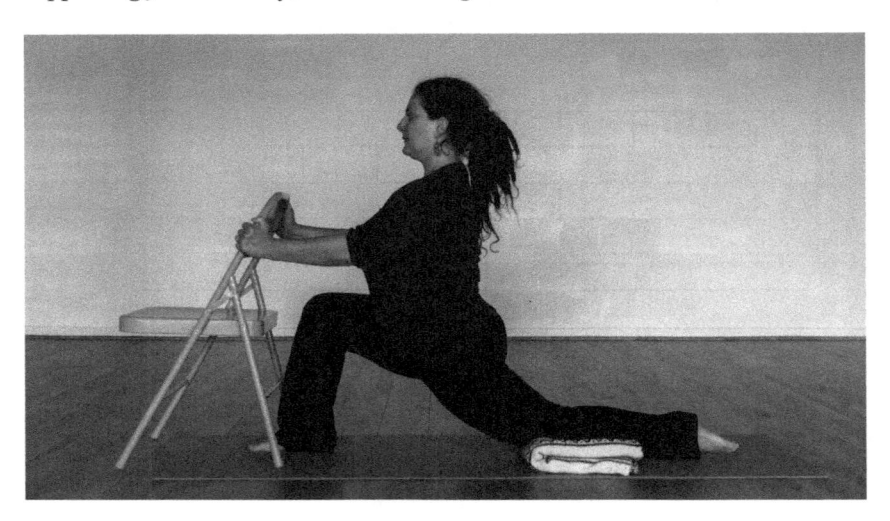

Figure 9.7 Low Lunge.

Note: Focus on lengthening hip flexors (iliopsoas, rectus femoris, TFL). Maintain stability of the back without collapse into excessive anterior tilt or lumbar extension (backbending); proprioceptive awareness of body position and slight engagement of the "core," including transverse abdominals, facilitate this stability.

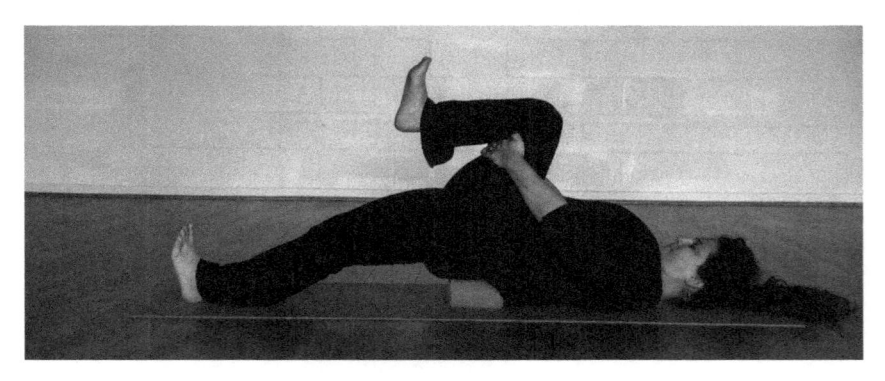

Figure 9.8 Supported Single-Leg Bridge.

Note: Focus on lengthening hip flexors (iliopsoas, rectus femoris, TFL). Place blankets or blocks under the sacrum as in supported bridge; hold one knee to the chest to decrease excessive backbending and lengthen the other leg along/toward the floor.

Setting the Stage for Well-Being 197

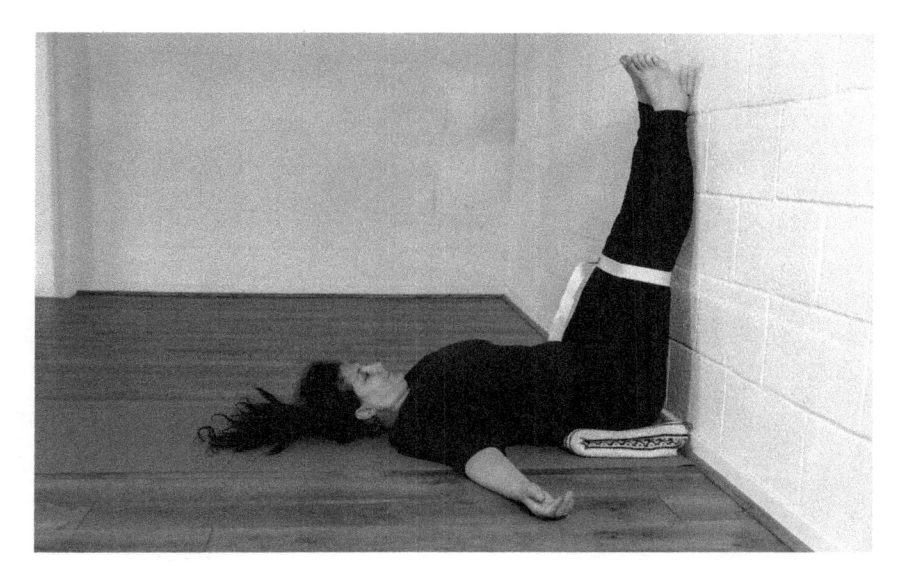

Figure 9.9 Legs Up the Wall.

Note: Focus on lengthening the hamstrings. With or without a blanket under the hips/sacrum; a belt around the thighs can help the muscles to relax.

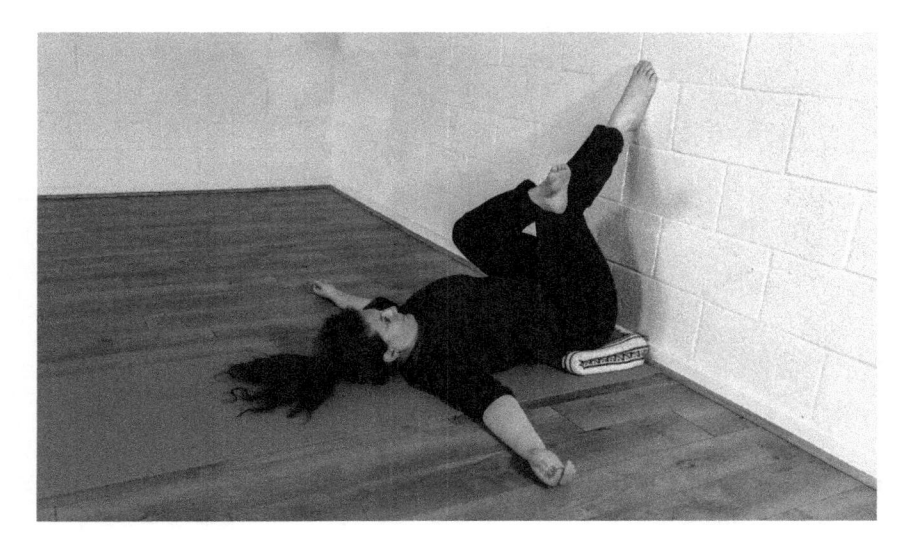

Figure 9.10 Figure-Four Legs Up the Wall.

Note: Focus on lengthening the hip rotators including the piriformis. Place one ankle above the opposite knee; either keep the other leg straightened up the wall or bend the knee to produce a comfortable degree of outer-hip sensation.

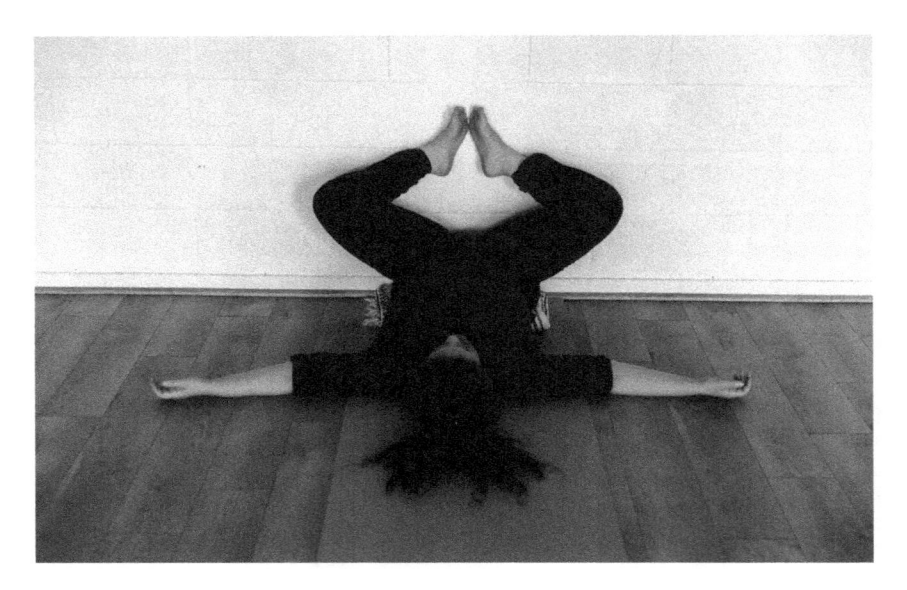

Figure 9.11 Bound-Angle Legs Up the Wall.

Note: Focus on lengthening the adductors.

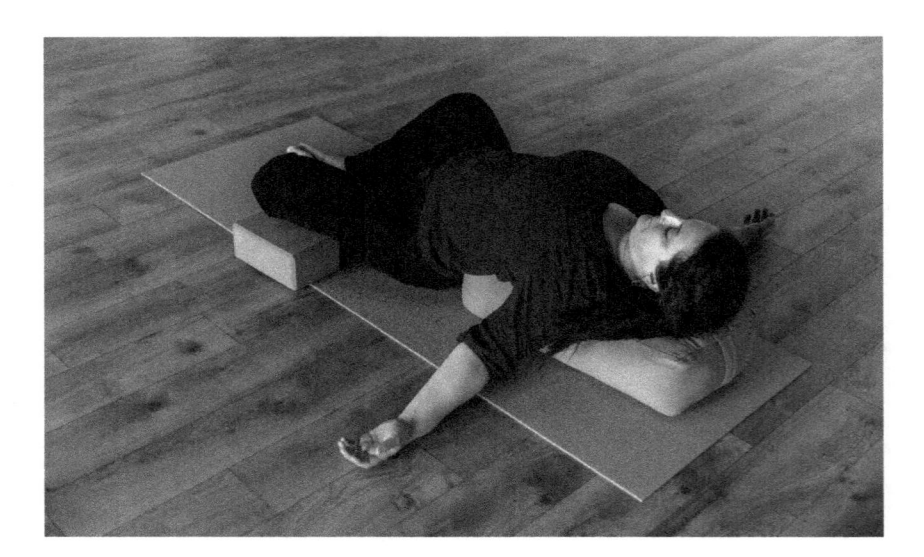

Figure 9.12 Supported Bound Angle.

Note: Focus on lengthening the adductors and chest, including the pectoralis muscles. Place blocks under the knees/thighs to allow the adductors to relax into length; support the spine and shoulder blades with a bolster.

Setting the Stage for Well-Being 199

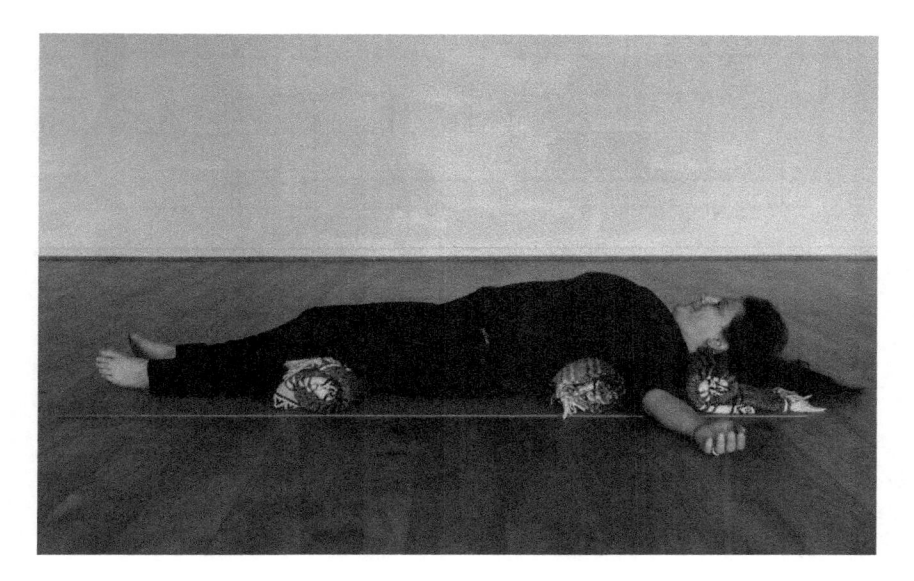

Figure 9.13 Mountain Brook.

Note: Focus on lengthening the pectoralis muscles. Roll blankets horizontally under the knees, at the bottom of or below the shoulder blades, and under the neck or base of the skull.

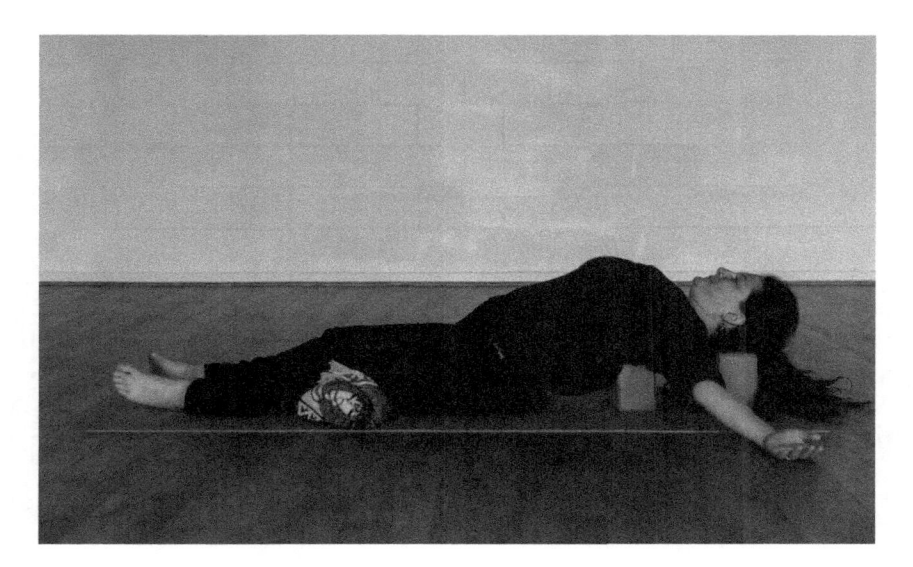

Figure 9.14 Supported Fish.

Note: Focus on lengthening the pectoralis muscles. Place blocks horizontally at the bottom of or slightly below the shoulder blades and under the head.

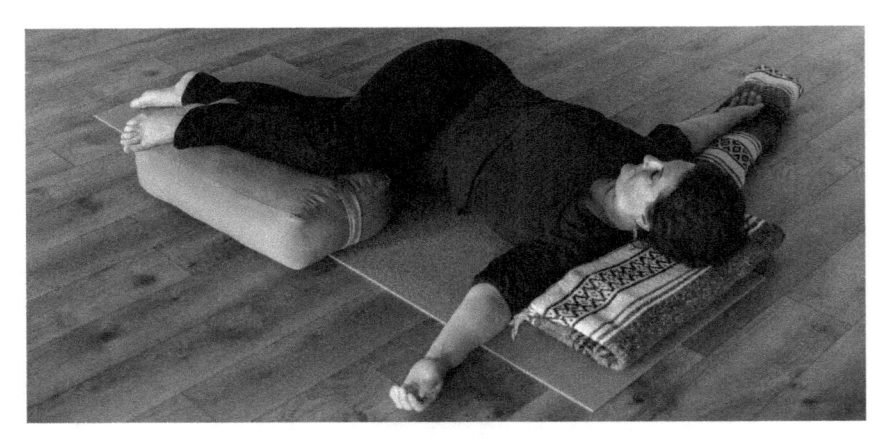

Figure 9.15 Supported Twist.

Note: Focus on lengthening the hip rotators and abductors (piriformis, glutes), trunk and abdominals, and chest. Aiming the nose straight up or toward the knees decreases stress on the neck and enhances lengthening of the pectoralis muscles.

Postures to Activate Weak/Inhibited Areas

These can be directed to engage muscles skillfully and promote stable, strong movement; support ease, comfort, and confidence; and improve proprioception. See Figures 9.16 to 9.22 for examples.

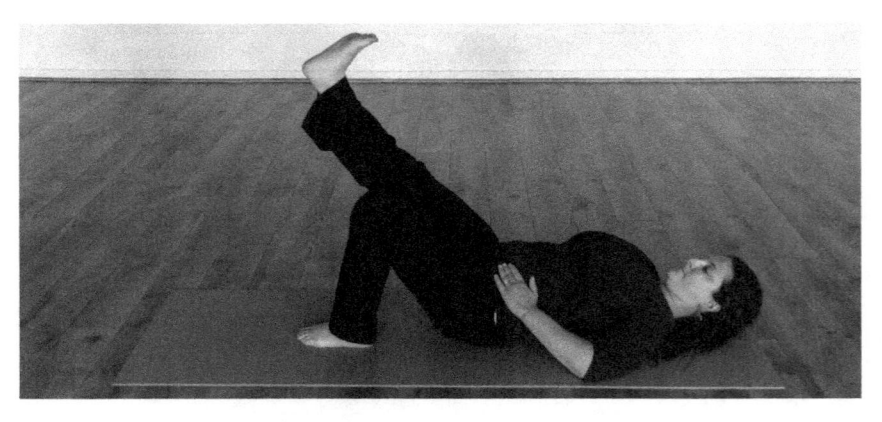

Figure 9.16 Supine Abdominal Engagement.

Note: With the pelvis in a neutral position (midway between anterior and posterior tilt with natural spinal curves), place the fingertips just inside the frontal pelvic bones. On exhalation, imagine drawing the two sit bones (ischial tuberosities) together; feel for the light engagement under the fingers. Increase the engagement by visualizing drawing the two pelvic bones together. If this can be done comfortably and with stability, straighten one leg toward the ceiling and slowly lift and lower it.

Setting the Stage for Well-Being 201

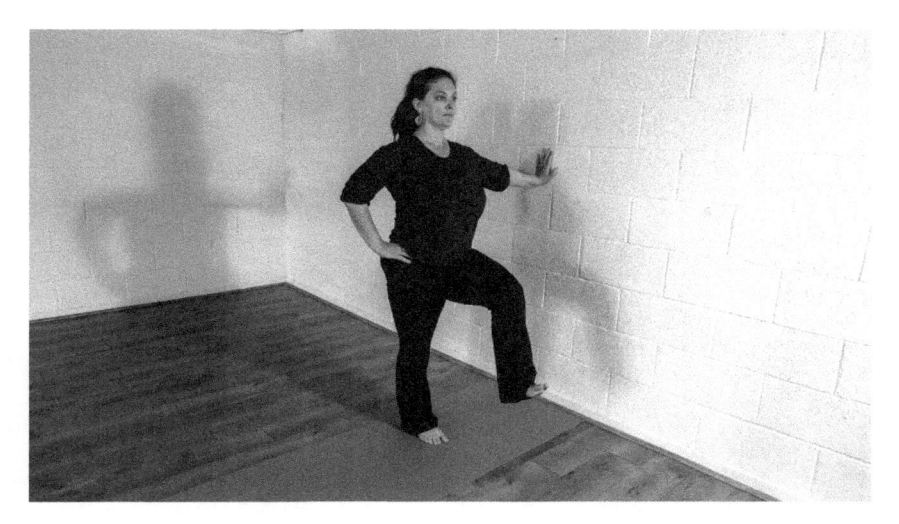

Figure 9.17 Single-Leg Standing.

Note: Focus on strengthening gluteus medius. Engage the glutes of the standing leg as if pressing a straight line down from outer hip to outer heel; imagine a second line drawing up from the inner arch of the foot, through the inner thigh and abdominals.

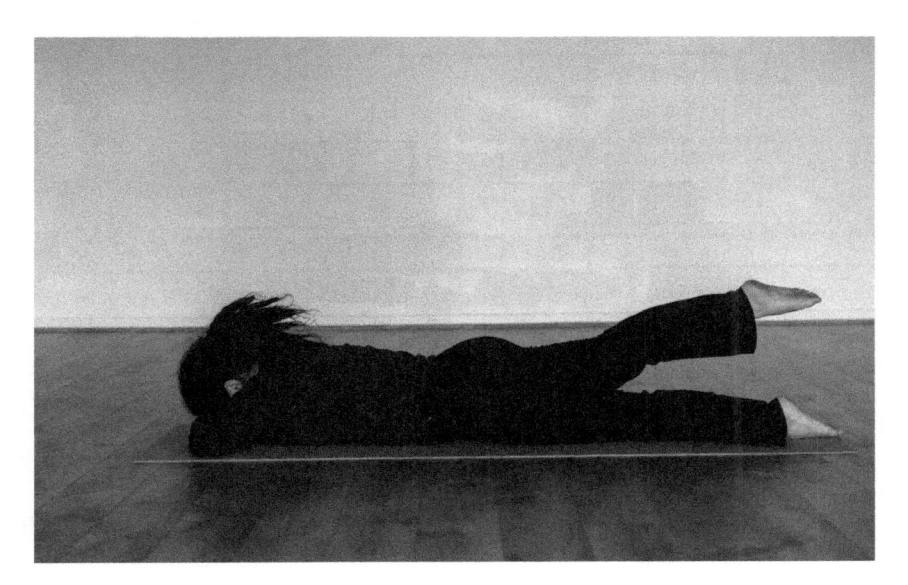

Figure 9.18 Half Locust—Lower Body.

Note: As in Figure 9.16, lightly engage the abdominals; then engage the glutes (visualize drawing tailbone toward heel) and lift the leg without tension in the neck or shoulders. Focus on strengthening the gluteus maximus.

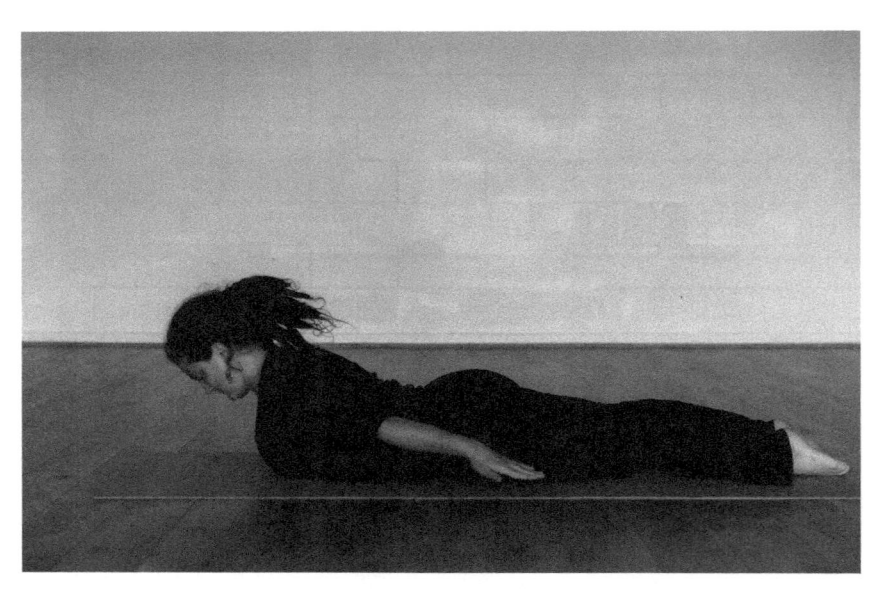

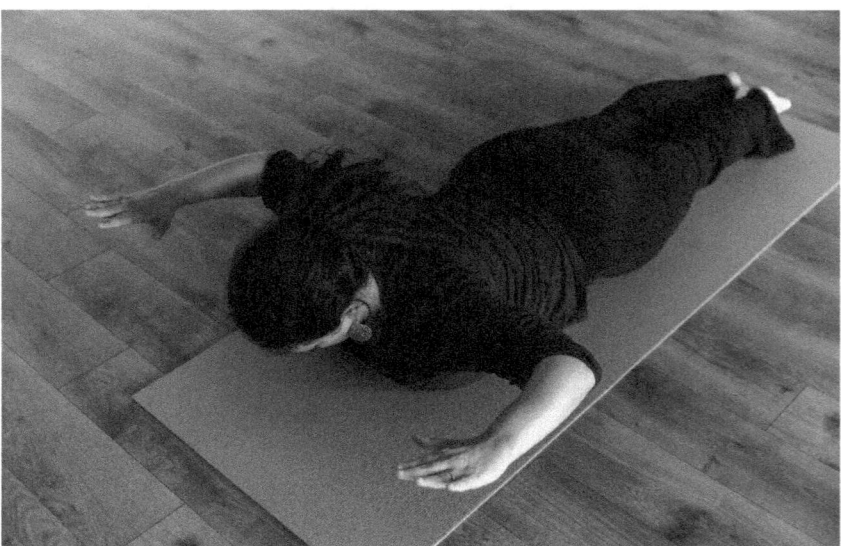

Figure 9.19 and Figure 9.20 Half Locust—Upper Body.

Notes: Focus on strengthening lower and middle trapezius. 1. Draw the shoulder blades together and down without excess tension in the neck, jaw, or shoulders; lift the head and upper body, adding the hands only if this can be done without neck or jaw tension. 2. With the elbows bent to 90 degrees, lift the hands and forearms, keeping the elbows on the ground; progress by lifting the elbows, feeling engagement between and below the shoulder blades. Add the arms, chest if no excess tension develops in the jaw or neck

Setting the Stage for Well-Being 203

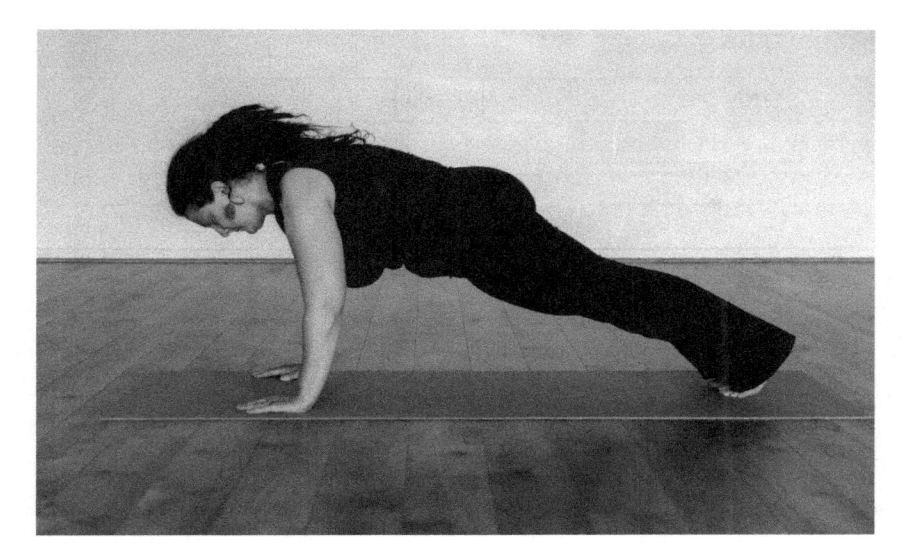

Figure 9.21 Plank.

Note: Focus on strengthening serratus anterior and "core." Press into the ground to lift the area between the shoulder blades; isometrically (without movement) drawing the hands toward each other and toward the feet can help engage the serratus and abdominal muscles.

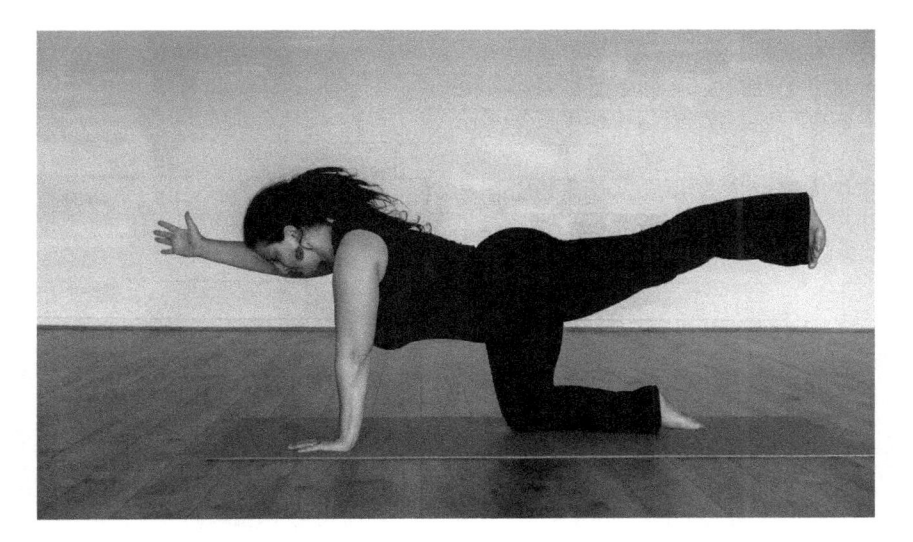

Figure 9.22 Bird Dog.

Note: Focus on strengthening serratus anterior, abdominals, and spinal muscles. From hands and knees, press the hands into the ground to lift the area between the shoulder blades; draw the hands isometrically toward each other and toward the knees, and lift opposite arm and leg.

Pranayama

Breathing practices can also be directed toward body-mind regulation. Like physical movement and position, purposefully directing the breath can cultivate sattva and the social engagement neural platform, leading to parasympathetic activation and relaxed body-mind states. Below are example breathing practices and their effects.

Slow-Paced Breath

Slowing the pace of respiration has been shown to positively affect stress, anger, depression, parasympathetic activation, cognitive control such as the ability to maintain focused attention, and emotional state.[6] A respiratory rate of 5 to 6 breaths a minute has these positive effects on physiology, emotion, and behavior in alignment with the attributes of the social engagement neural platform.[7]

Diaphragmatic and Three-Part Breath

Diaphragmatic breath has been shown to have combined effects for improved attention and affect and relaxed physiological states.[8]

> **Practice 9.3 Diaphragmatic Breathing Method: Dirgha Pranayama**
>
> Start supine with knees bent and feet on the floor, or in constructive rest from Figure 9.2.
>
> - Place one hand on the abdomen and the other on the chest.
> - When you inhale, notice whether you can feel the abdomen rising up into that hand. As you exhale, the abdomen rests back down toward the floor. Can you allow the movement to be primarily in the abdomen and less in the chest? Repeat this pattern for 3 to 5 rounds of breath.
> - Place the hands on the side ribs. As you inhale, continue to allow the abdomen to move up toward the ceiling while moving the ribs

> out to the sides. On each inhalation the abdomen rises and the side ribs expand; on each exhalation they settle back to their original positions. Repeat for 3 to 5 rounds of breath.
> - Place a hand on the chest and the abdomen again. As you inhale, feel the abdomen rise up into your hand and the ribs expand to the sides but now also allow the chest to rise up into your hand at the top of the breath. Exhale and notice how the body settles back to its original position. Repeat for 3 to 5 rounds of breath.
> - Continue the full breath for 5 to 10 minutes, if it is comfortable.

Breath With Sound: Ujjayi and Bhramari

Ujjayi breathing involves creating airway resistance by gently contracting the laryngeal muscles during both inhalation and exhalation. The resistance is thought to be beneficial for slowing the breath; a rate of 4 to 9 breaths per minute, considerably slower than the generally cited average of 12 to 20 breaths per minute for adults, supports parasympathetic activation.[9] Laryngeal constriction may also influence vagal afferents, promoting a parasympathetic response. This activation of the social engagement neural platform

> ### Practice 9.4 Ujjayi Pranayama Method
>
> Ujjayi can be added to the diaphragmatic three-part breath.
>
> - Put a hand in front of your mouth as if holding a small mirror. Exhale through the mouth, creating a slight contracture in the throat as if you were fogging the mirror. Continue to breathe in through the nose and out through the mouth, making the mirror-fogging sound as you exhale. Repeat this pattern 3 to 5 times.
> - Continue, but now keep your mouth closed as you exhale, continuing to make the sound.
> - As you feel comfortable, add the sound to the inhalation, too.
>
> Creating a smooth ujjayi breath through the course of a complete respiration requires time and practice. Avoiding strain is much more important than creating a particular sound or volume.

results in a combined physiological and psychological state of calm alertness, also characteristic of sattvic qualities like clarity. Ujjayi breath is often called "victorious breath," as it helps to calm and steady the mind—to achieve victory over its fluctuations. It is also known as "ocean breath" because the sound produced is similar to that of ocean waves.

The word *bhramari* means "bee." This pranayama, which invites the inwardly focused gaze of *pratyahara,* or sensory withdrawal, has been shown to be beneficial for symptoms of anxiety. It also supports activation of the parasympathetic nervous system for physiological relaxation and restoration as seen through cardiovascular parameters such as blood pressure, heart rate variability, and heart rate.[10]

Practice 9.5 Bhramari Pranayama Method

- Sit comfortably and allow a few deep, slow breaths through the nostrils, practicing three-part diaphragmatic breath.
- When you are ready to begin, inhale through the nose. Keep the mouth closed as you exhale, creating a buzzing hum. You can bring the hum's vibration into the chest, throat, mouth, or head.
- Try to breathe at a rate between 4 and 6 breaths per minute.
- Alternatively, experiment with different pitches and with further blocking off external stimuli by gently pressing the fingers over the eyes and/or ears.

Alternate- and Unilateral-Nostril Breathing

Alternate-nostril breath, sometimes referred to as *nadi shodhana,* has been shown to activate the parasympathetic nervous system as demonstrated by measures of heart rate and blood pressure. This type of pranayama also affects cognitive processes for improved sustained attention.[11] Left-nostril breathing increases parasympathetic activity, including increased heart rate variability.[12] Right-nostril breathing has been shown to increase sympathetic activity.[13] These different effects indicate that we can tailor alternate- or left-nostril breathing to activate the parasympathetic nervous system and right-nostril breathing for sympathetic activation. Different yogic schools of thought suggest various patterns for encouraging particular effects.

Practice 9.6 Alternate-Nostril Pranayama Method

- Start with three-part diaphragmatic breath.
- Bring the right hand to the nose. Fold the index and middle finger to the palm so that the thumb rests on the right nostril and the ring finger rests on the left. Gently press the right nostril closed and exhale through the left; inhale through the left nostril. Close the left nostril and exhale through the right; inhale through the right nostril. Continue switching sides after the inhalation for 5 to 10 minutes, ending with an exhalation through the left nostril.
- Alternatively, experiment with using your left hand to block the nostrils, gently drawing the chin toward the chest, and/or resting the index and middle fingers between the eyebrows.

Meditation

Meditation practices are powerful ways to promote body-mind regulation. (See Chapter 8 for references and more detailed descriptions of these mechanisms.) In addition to those below, see Practices 1.2 (p. 28) and 2.2 (p. 44), respectively, for explorations of connection to awareness and to sustained meaning, purpose, and harmony.

Loving-Kindness

In the Yoga Sutras, verse 1.33 emphasizes the cultivation of friendliness and compassion, sometimes interpreted as loving-kindness. We can consider this type of meditation as a way of strengthening neural pathways that promote positive mental states and prosocial behavioral attributes for well-being. I have adapted Jack Kornfield's loving-kindness meditation slightly for use with clients.[14] In my experience, people find it most difficult to cultivate positive emotions toward themselves, so I usually begin by having the person visualize a person, animal, or place for which they feel love and/or a positive connection. For many clients this is most easily felt in connection with a pet.

> **Practice 9.7 Meditation on Loving-Kindness**
>
> - Visualize a person or animal to whom you feel connected and/or a sense of love for. Notice how that love and connection feels in your body. Sit with these feelings for a moment, then offer the person or animal this prayer or intention:
>   - May you be filled with loving-kindness. May you be safe from inner and outer harm. May your mind and body be filled with ease. May you be well and happy.
>   - Feel the giving (and perhaps the loved one's receipt) of this intention.
>   - Pause at the end of each sentence or at the end of the full intention to experience this giving and receiving.
> - Next, visualize others you love and feel connected to. Repeat the intention statements, again pausing to feel the experience of giving and these others receiving.
> - Visualize someone with whom you have had stress or trouble and offer this intention to them. Repeat the intention statements and pause to feel the experience of giving and this person receiving.
> - Finally, offer these words to yourself. Repeat the intention statements and pause to feel the experience of giving to and receiving in yourself.

Mantra or Affirmation

The loving-kindness meditation (Practice 9.7) is a kind of affirmation or *mantra* practice, as it involves the repetition of a phrase. I find developing any kind of affirmational word or phrase to be useful in promoting the foundation of sattva guna and body-mind regulation.

With clients I often start with a discussion on the intention they would like to cultivate to feel safe and connected; they then reflect on a word, image, or affirmation that embodies this feeling for them. Some people work with pets such as birds, dogs, or horses, or with natural images like an ocean or forest. Others create a word or phrase such as "home," "peace," "may I be filled with love," or "may my heart and mind be calm and at ease." The client then spends 5 to 15 minutes focusing on this image or word(s), allowing other thoughts, emotions, and sensations to arise and pass away and simply bringing attention back to the intention when distraction inevitably arises.

Although we may think of meditation as requiring a specific formal posture, I often consider ways in which the practice can be incorporated into daily life, for example, before bed or during a commute. Sitting, lying supine, standing, and walking are traditional possibilities for meditation postures, but a less formal practice supports the development of a habit and illustrates to clients how easily mindful intention can become part of their routines without devoting extra time to it.

Body Scan and Visualization

Chapter 1 includes a meditation on connection and unity with awareness (see Practice 1.2, p. 28) that incorporates a body scan and intention offering to each part of the body. This type of practice can be used to cultivate sattva and body-mind regulation, and Practice 9.8 illustrates another way of strengthening sattva guna and body-mind regulation through a body scan.

Practice 9.8 Body Scan

Find a comfortable position, supine if possible.
- Allow the body to settle and the breath to become effortless and soft.
- Invite an image or memory that brings a sense of peace, love, connection, or ease. As you stay with this image or memory, notice where in your body you feel these sensations. Notice their qualities, textures, and/or colors—maybe lightness, expansion, groundedness, and so on.
- Notice where you feel these sensations most strongly in your body and focus your attention there. Then, offer this feeling to each part of your body in turn (begin the scan anywhere but work methodically through the body):
    ○ head, face, throat, and neck;
    ○ right and left shoulders, right arm to fingertips, left arm to fingertips;
    ○ chest and area around the heart, abdomen, sides of the torso and back of the body, pelvis—front, left and right sides, back; and
    ○ right and left hip, right thigh to foot, left thigh to foot.
- Notice arising thoughts, emotions, or beliefs and offer this feeling to each.

Practice 9.9 Reflections on Spiritual and Eudaimonic Well-Being

Use these practices for journaling or meditation that supports spiritual and eudaimonic well-being for body-mind regulation, sattva guna, and the positive psychological and prosocial qualities of the social engagement neural platform.

Meaning and Purpose

- What brings meaning or purpose to your life? What has been meaningful in your past, is meaningful now, and what do you feel will be meaningful in your future? What do you consider to be your purpose?
- Write a statement (one to three sentences) about your meaning and purpose.
- When you are in alignment with your meaning and purpose, what do you notice? You might consider a time in your past when you felt connected to this dharma.
  - What kinds of thoughts, emotions, and beliefs were present? How and where did you feel them in your body? What people or situations surrounded you? What kinds of actions were you taking at this time?
  - How does this meaning and purpose relate to a situation you are currently experiencing? How might this guidance help you to understand or work with the situation in a beneficial way?

Virtues

- Consider certain virtues as in Practice 9.1 (p. 186).
- What virtues continue to show up as important to you?
- How do you want to embody that virtue or virtues in your interactions with yourself? With others? With life situations?

Personal Connectedness/Self-Actualization/Authenticity/Personal Expressiveness

- Reflect on what you consider to be your strengths and gifts.
- Consider also the perception of your weaknesses. Are there ways in which these weaknesses are also strengths? How have they helped you?

- What would it mean to appreciate *all* of yourself—not just gifts, but the way even your weaknesses have served you? How can perceived weaknesses become part of your gifts?
- Consider a time when you faced adversity and it became an opportunity for growth, how your gifts and weaknesses helped you to grow into your full potential in the situation.
- How have your life circumstances been opportunities for growth, transformation, and living to your full potential?

Social Relationships

- What does it mean to have positive, meaningful relationships?
- If it is helpful, consider one such relationship and reflect on why it is a meaningful one.
- What does it mean to you to feel connected to another person, to trust and to have empathy and compassion for another person? What does it mean to receive connection, trust, empathy, and compassion?

Existential/Transcendental Connection

- What does it mean to connect to something outside yourself? To life? To the environment? To something greater?
- When connected in this way, what qualities do you notice? Lightness? Expansiveness? Love? How do you notice those qualities in your body, thoughts, and emotions?
- What would it be like to relate to your life from the standpoint of this connection?

Conclusion

The practices of yoga, which include yama, niyama, asana, pranayama, and meditation, can be used together to create body-mind regulation, cultivate sattva guna, and activate the social engagement neural platform through the koshas and biopsychosocial-spiritual model. Physically (annamaya), we cultivate and support relaxed physiological states through parasympathetic activation, healthy interoceptive processes, improved body awareness, and proprioception. Energetically (pranamaya), we support qualities and experiences such as clarity, luminosity, vitality, calm, ease, buoyancy, expansiveness, and stability. In the realm of mind and emotion (manomaya), we can support mood regulation, positive psychological and emotional states, and improved cognitive and attentional control and regulation. For supporting wisdom and discrimination (vijnanamaya), we cultivate the ability to notice habits of relating to the body, mind, others, and life itself. By recognizing how our tendencies either create suffering or alleviate it we can begin to explore non-judgmental observation. In the realm of bliss or awe (anandamaya), we support experiences of spiritual and eudaimonic well-being.

Notes

1. Gupta, B. (2006). Bhagavad Gītā as duty and virtue ethics: Some reflections. *Journal of Religious Ethics*, 34(3), 373–395.
2. Cottingham, J. T., Porges, S. W., & Richmond, K. (1988). Shifts in pelvic inclination angle and parasympathetic tone produced by Rolfing soft tissue manipulation. *Physical Therapy*, 68(9), 1364–1370.; Cottingham, J. T., Porges, S. W., & Lyon, T. (1988). Effects of soft tissue mobilization (Rolfing pelvic lift) on parasympathetic tone in two age groups. *Physical Therapy*, 68(3), 352–356.
3. Shafir, T., Tsachor, R. P., & Welch, K. B. (2016). Emotion regulation through movement: Unique sets of movement characteristics are associated with and enhance basic emotions. *Frontiers in Psychology*, 6, 2030.
4. Farb, N., Daubenmier, J., Price, C. J., Gard, T., Kerr, C., Dunn, B. D., ... & Mehling, W. E. (2015). Interoception, contemplative practice, and health. *Frontiers in Psychology*, 6, 763; Fiori, F., Aglioti, S. M., & David, N. (2017). Interactions between body and social awareness in yoga. *Journal of Alternative and Complementary Medicine*, 23(3), 227–233; Haase, L., Stewart, J. L., Youssef, B., May, A. C., Isakovic, S., Simmons, A. N., ... & Paulus, M. P. (2016). When the brain does not adequately feel the body: Links between low resilience and interoception. *Biological Psychology*, 113, 37–45.
5. For more on the Janda philosophy and its application, see: Page, P., Frank, C. C., & Lardner, R. (2010). *Assessment and treatment of muscle imbalance: The Janda approach*. Champaign, IL: Human Kinetics.
6. For references and more information, see: Brown, R. P., Gerbarg, P. L., & Muench, F. (2013). Breathing practices for treatment of psychiatric and stress-related medical conditions. *Psychiatric Clinics of North America*, 36(1), 121–140; Mason, H., Vandoni, M., deBarbieri, G., Codrons, E., Ugargol, V., & Bernardi, L. (2013). Cardiovascular and respiratory effect of yogic slow breathing in the yoga beginner: What is the best approach? *Evidence-Based Complementary and Alternative Medicine*, 2013, 1–7.
7. Ibid.
8. Ma, X., Yue, Z.-Q., Gong, Z.-Q., Zhang, H., Duan, N.-Y., Shi, Y.-T., ... Li, Y.-F. (2017). The effect of diaphragmatic breathing on attention, negative affect and stress in healthy adults. *Frontiers in Psychology*, 8. https://doi.org/10.3389/fpsyg.2017.00874
9. Brown, R. P., & Gerbarg, P. L. (2005). Sudarshan kriya yogic breathing in the treatment of stress, anxiety, and depression: Part II—Clinical applications and guidelines. *Journal of Alternative and Complementary Medicine*, 11(4), 711–717; Brown, R. P., &

Gerbarg, P. L. (2005). *Sudarshan kriya* yogic breathing in the treatment of stress, anxiety, and depression: Part I—Neurophysiologic model. *Journal of Alternative and Complementary Medicine, 11*(1), 189–201; Mason et al., Cardiovascular and respiratory effect of yogic slow breathing in the yoga beginner.

10. Telles, S., & Naveen, K. (2008). Voluntary breath regulation in yoga: Its relevance and physiological effects. *Biofeedback, 36*(2), 70–73; Kuppusamy, M., Kamaldeen, D., Pitani, R., & Amaldas, J. (2016). Immediate effects of Bhramari pranayama on resting cardiovascular parameters in healthy adolescents. *Journal of Clinical and Diagnostic Research: JCDR, 10*(5), CC17; Nivethitha, L., Manjunath, N., & Mooventhan, A. (2017). Heart rate variability changes during and after the practice of bhramari pranayama. *International Journal of Yoga, 10*(2), 99–102.
11. Telles & Naveen, Voluntary breath regulation in yoga; Balkrishna, A. (2014). Blood pressure and heart rate variability during yoga-based alternate nostril breathing practice and breath awareness. *Medical Science Monitor Basic Research, 20*, 184–193; Bhavanani, A., Pushpa, D., Ramanathan, M., & Balaji, R. (2014). Differential effects of uninostril and alternate nostril pranayamas on cardiovascular parameters and reaction time. *International Journal of Yoga, 7*(1), 60; Naik, G. S., Gaur, G. S., & Pal, G. K. (2018). Effect of modified slow breathing exercise on perceived stress and basal cardiovascular parameters. *International Journal of Yoga, 11*(1), 53–58; Raghuraj, P., & Telles, S. (2008). Immediate effect of specific nostril manipulating yoga breathing practices on autonomic and respiratory variables. *Applied Psychophysiology and Biofeedback, 33*(2), 65–75; Telles, S., Singh, N., & Puthige, R. (2013). Changes in P300 following alternate nostril yoga breathing and breath awareness. *BioPsychoSocial Medicine, 7*(1), 11. https://doi.org/10.1186/1751-0759-7-11; Sinha, A. N., Deepak, D., & Singh Gusain, V. (2013). Assessment of the effects of pranayama/alternate nostril breathing on the parasympathetic nervous system in young adults. *Journal of Clinical and Diagnostic Research, 7*(5), 821–823.
12. Telles & Naveen, Voluntary breath regulation in yoga; Bhavanani, Pushpa, Ramanathan, & Balaji, Differential effects of uninostril and alternate nostril pranayamas; Pal, G., Agarwal, A., Karthik, S., Pal, P., & Nanda, N. (2014). Slow yogic breathing through right and left nostril influences sympathovagal balance, heart rate variability, and cardiovascular risks in young adults. *North American Journal of Medical Sciences, 6*(3), 145. https://doi.org/10.4103/1947-2714.128477; Raghuraj & Telles, Immediate effect of specific nostril manipulating yoga breathing practices.
13. Telles & Naveen, Voluntary breath regulation in yoga; Bhavanani, Pushpa, Ramanathan, & Balaji, Differential effects of uninostril and alternate nostril pranayamas; Pal, Agarwal, Karthik, Pal, & Nanda, Slow yogic breathing through right and left nostril; Raghuraj & Telles, Immediate effect of specific nostril manipulating yoga breathing practices.
14. https://jackkornfield.com/meditation-on-lovingkindness. Kornfield's phrasing, in turn, is based on traditional Buddhist meditations.

Cultivating Healthy Sensitivity

Interoceptive Skills and Discriminative Wisdom

The practices in this chapter build on those in Chapter 9, which focuses on the cultivation of sattva guna and body-mind regulation. This foundation of safety, peace, relaxation, and regulatory capacity is essential to support deep inquiry into habits of relating to stimuli of the body, mind, and environment. Yoga's practices include those that support self-reflection and self-study for transformation to alleviate suffering.

The practices here are meant to encourage a sense of curiosity and compassionate, nonjudgmental exploration of oneself. From a neurophysiological perspective, these practices build healthy interoceptive and proprioceptive skills to help us to recognize relationships among physical sensations, mental constructs, and relationships to others and life circumstances. From a yogic perspective, they cultivate discriminative wisdom to help us recognize the difference between the body-mind-environment and our essential nature as awareness. Samkhya concepts including purusha, prakriti, the gunas, aspects of the mind, as well as the koshas and prana vayus (Chapters 3 to 5) inform such inquiry.

Building interoception, proprioception, and discriminative wisdom helps us to develop more accurate, flexible abilities to evaluate and interpret sensation. We are invited into a process of reflection, self-discovery, and transformation of habitual reactions to support improved well-being.

Yama and Niyama

Chapter 9 describes how ethical inquiry provides insight into living in alignment with one's values to fulfill dharma and realize eudaimonic well-being.

These practices use the ethical principles of yoga to support body-mind regulation, sattva guna, and the social engagement neural platform. Building on this foundation, we can use the yamas and niyamas to cultivate sensitivity. The essential ethical principle of svadhyaya (Chapter 5) invites us to embody or entextualize yoga to enter into deep self-inquiry and self-study. Svadhyaya is vital to the next stage of practice, in which we reflect on relationships to body, mind, and environmental stimuli from a perspective of curiosity, nonjudgmental observation, and compassion.

Practices for Svadhyaya

Most of the practices in this book are forms of svadhyaya. They support the development of curiosity to help us to:

- recognize habitual patterns of reaction and relationships to body-mind-environmental stimuli (see Practices 1.1, p. 19; 3.1, p. 56; 3.2, p. 65; and 4.1, p. 75);
- realize our essential nature as awareness (see Practices 1.2, p. 28; 3.1, p. 56; 3.2, p. 65; and 5.2, p. 102);
- reflect on ethical principles (see Practices 2.1, p. 33; 9.1, p. 186; and 9.2, p. 187) that also support the actualization of dharma and its harmony in relating to ourselves, others, and life (see Practices 2.1, p. 33; and 2.2, p. 44);
- develop discernment between the body-mind-environment and awareness (see Practices 3.1, p. 56; 3.2, p. 65; and 4.1, p. 75); and
- reflect on eudaimonic and spiritual well-being (see Practice 6.1, p. 124).

All ethical inquiry can be beneficial for this process of self-study, but particular principles or attributes support this compassionate, nonjudgmental reflection. Curiosity, kindness, nonharming, contentment, truth, acceptance, and patience are a few examples that can be explored through practices such as the golden mean (Practice 9.1, p. 186), reflective questions (Practice 9.2, p. 187), and relationship to dharma (Practice 2.1, p. 33).

> ### Practice 10.1 Reflections on Yamas/Niyamas
>
> Other reflections on these ethical principles might include the following.
>
> - What does the concept mean to you? How has it shown up in your life? How would you like this concept to be in your life? How can

you support the development of this principle in a way that aids your well-being? How can this principle inform the way you relate to body, mind, and environmental stimuli? How can this principle support healthy interactions with yourself, others, and life circumstances? What kind of movement, breath, visualization, or affirmation might help you to embody and "become" this principle?
- Reflect and journal on the concept. You might also create meditations or movement practices for insight into how the ethical principles relate to yourself and support your well-being.

Clinical Example

"Michele" reported frustration with years of low back and sacroiliac joint pain. She felt unable to trust her body because she could not participate in work and social activities as she previously had, or in the ways she wished she could. Her pain often created an experience of feeling unsupported in life, as Michele felt that others did not understand her pain or loss of function or were not able to really hear her concerns.

We discussed her frustration, mistrust of the body, and lack of support. Michele also expressed difficulty listening to the needs of her body—she feared that this would further prevent her from enjoying or participating in life.

We decided to work with intentions of support and inner strength, patience, and kindness. She journaled on the excess, deficiency, and mean of each concept as well as her tendencies on the continuum. Michele considered times in her life when she felt inner strength, patience, and kindness. She also thought about when she had exhibited these qualities in relationships with others and under what circumstances. She explored what these three principles would feel like in her body. For Michele, inner strength was reflected in an image of a redwood tree extending through the entire back of her body. Patience took the shape of observing the slow growth of the tree. She felt kindness throughout the body as an expansive quality of resting on the tree, soaking in the sun and the nourishment of the earth. Practicing supported bound angle (see Figure 9.12), supported bridge (see Figure 9.3), tree, and warrior I helped to strengthen these images and experiences for her.

With these practices as a foundation, Michele made a commitment to explore each day what would happen if she listened to her body. She would ask what her body needed, particularly when rest or activity would be useful.

When she felt frustrated with her body, Michele could do the imagery practice and decide whether to include the physical practices. Over time, she found greater kindness and receptivity to her body's signals. She also experienced less frustration and more inner strength.

The asana, pranayama, and meditation practices below are provided in this context of the compassionate, reflective inquiry of svadhyaya. The capacity for imbuing curiosity with kindness and compassion is important to a transformative process as we dive into deep reflection and exploration of ourselves and our relationships.

Asana as Svadhyaya and Inquiry

Improving Proprioception

Healthy proprioception includes accurately discerning where the body is in space both in static positions and during movement. This mindful awareness of position supports easier, more functional movement.

Altered proprioception and its potential adverse effects can appear in a number of ways. Someone might stand or move in a way that creates patterns of stress or strain that affect range of motion, producing compressive forces on the joints or soft tissue structures and even altering muscular recruitment. For example, habitually standing with an excessive pelvic tilt (in either direction) could contribute to muscle imbalances, including altered length or activation, as discussed in Chapter 9. An excessive anterior pelvic tilt often co-occurs with a shortening and/or tightness of the iliopsoas and weakness/inhibition of the transverse abdominals and gluteus maximus, whereas excessive posterior tilt often co-occurs with shortened hamstrings and weak or inhibited gluteus maximus.

In cases of joint instability, accurate perception of joint position is lacking and neuromotor control is altered. The person might overextend their joints or move past the optimal range of motion for an activity. As above, this overextension often co-occurs with altered muscular recruitment and engagement patterns. The knees may overextend in standing postures like mountain or warriors, for instance, or the elbows may overextend in weight-bearing on the hands and knees. Someone might also move excessively in one part of the body rather than evenly distributing the motion, creating an unhealthy fulcrum. This can be seen in forward folds with an overly rounded spine or in backbends that extend only the cervical rather than the cervical and thoracic spine.

Sensory loss resulting from neurological conditions such as multiple sclerosis may result in an inability to feel where the body is in space. Chronic, persistent pain is also associated with changes in sensory and motor function resulting in altered proprioception and muscular activation patterns. Chronic pain may even result in distorted body image, where the painful body part seems larger, nonexistent, or withered, or the person ignores the area or experiences it differently from other parts of the body (e.g., as a different color).[1]

These deficits in proprioception can contribute to loss of function, discomfort, and loss of ease with movement or in static positions. Working with both proprioceptive and interoceptive skills helps clients to "re-map" the body—to normalize body image and connect to sensation in healthy ways. We can also promote optimal muscular engagement patterns for easier movement. Chapters 7 and 8 discuss the importance of healthy interoceptive and proprioceptive skills in relation to self-regulation, resilience, and empathy.[2]

There is no single correct alignment for all bodies. When considering practices to improve proprioceptive awareness, it is important to emphasize that everyone has a unique optimal alignment. The most ideal practices to create easeful, functional movement differ from person to person. Rather than offering an objective, rigid idea of posture and alignment, my intention is to facilitate a body-mind connection that creates an experience of support, openness, or lightness, optimizing stability and ease.

To develop this self-inquiry and exploration for proprioception, I ask clients simple questions as they move into or hold postures:

- How does this feel in the right leg, low back, etc., or in your whole body?
- Does your body feel supported, open, light, grounded, easeful, stable…in this position or movement? (Choose one or two of these qualities.)
- Does this posture create greater connection to your body as a whole/to this part of your body?

Often, when I introduce a new way of standing or moving, I meet with resistance. Even when a new pattern feels stronger, more stable, or more open, the client may worry that they are making an extreme change. In these cases, when the client is able to do so easily, I have them look at a mirror as a visual aid. Their minds rest easier when they see that the new position is actually not extreme. Once they see their balanced posture in the mirror, I ask clients to close their eyes (assuming the balance allows this) and perform a body scan to learn the inner sensation of the new posture. Through this practice, people create an inner blueprint to find the positions that create easier, more functional movement. The mirror comes with a downside if the person uses it for self-judgment, but it can be incredibly helpful for some people at certain moments in their practices.

Clinical Example

"Cheryl" experienced low back pain that was worsened by standing and back-bending. She often felt unstable or unsupported in her body. In standing, she demonstrated an increased anterior pelvic tilt and lumbar lordosis, and her knees tended toward overextension. She also exhibited this tendency to collapse into an anterior tilt and extension in her low back with postures like plank and warriors.

We used a mirror to explore different standing postures and find a neutral position for Cheryl's pelvis and back where she felt connected to her body as well as light, expansive, grounded, and stable. She reported that this position felt like an extremely rounded back, but the mirror demonstrated to her that she looked balanced and not at all rounded.

Cheryl then closed her eyes to remember this position, connecting to the inner sensations involved with her body being there. This allowed her to create a new template of standing to explore throughout her day. She learned about her habits of standing, to sense when she moved away from this feeling of lightness and stability, and how to return to it. We used a mirror to explore other postures. Cheryl looked at the position of her back and explored various alignments in warrior II and plank, for example, until she found those that created the same experience of connection, lightness, and groundedness. She closed her eyes to remember the position so that she could practice it without a mirror. Over time, Cheryl developed greater accuracy at finding a balanced position in all of her activities. Her low back discomfort decreased, and she was able to find more ease in movement and throughout her day.

Without a mirror, Cheryl had felt that these new positions created a gross misalignment, but the mirror helped her to see that these new postures looked balanced and enabled her to settle into a new template for movement.

I often use this method for clients who tend to over-round the low back when seated. For such people, more neutral spinal positions often feel overly extended and like they are "sticking their butt out," but the mirror lets them visually confirm that they are in neutral so the mind can inform the body to relax into the new posture.

There are other ways to guide proprioceptive experiences. Using visual or tactile cues, I might have clients assess where their body is in space and guide them to finding postures that create ease and stability. For example, someone in warrior II can find an easeful arm position, mindfully look at this alignment, then close her eyes and remember the position. A more tactile person might place her hands on her pelvis and move through an anterior and posterior tilt in standing to find the pelvic position that creates stability and ease. Whether using a mirror or another visual cue or exploring in a tactile way, once the new position is learned with one of these external aids I have clients close their eyes to imprint the new habit in the body.

Yet another way of working with proprioception is a basic body scan, in any posture, for noticing key landmarks with eyes both open and closed: the crown of the head, neck, shoulders, arms, torso, hips, knees, and feet. This can help people connect to the body both interoceptively and proprioceptively and learn how to hold positions and move with greater ease and stability.

Kosha Meditation

Another body-based practice I use to cultivate svadhyaya is a kosha reflection and meditation done in an asana. This practice is intended to provide the opportunity for insight into how movement and/or body positions affect the layers of experience from gross to subtle. Such meditations may also build proprioceptive and interoceptive skills.

We can draw attention to specific areas of the body with postures, then shift the focus from physical sensation to the recognition of energy, thoughts, and emotions, and finally to an ability to observe these sensations in the presence of steadfast contentment. Any posture can be used as a foundation for inquiry. For example, supported fish (see Figure 9.14) can be used to bring attention to the chest and shoulders, or a seated forward fold to explore the hamstrings and back of the body. This practice is intended to help people learn to articulate feelings and sensations in a nonjudgmental, noncognitive, abstract manner. (See Figure 7.1, p. 145 for a representation of this process of moving from emotion or behavior to underlying feeling.) I find this practice to be helpful in developing a shared language with clients. I learn how the person perceives and articulates sensations, and the client gains insight into the relationship between movement and effects along the koshas.

If a client has difficulty identifying and articulating sensation, I offer adjectives to help. My yoga therapy teacher, Julie Wilcox,[3] taught me that we gather as much information from the descriptors that resonate with someone's experiences as from those that do not. If the adjective I offer does not reflect the client's experience, they learn what is *not* true for them. They also learn that they can express themselves, will be listened to, and will have the opportunity to explore what *would* be most true for them. This exploration requires open-mindedness from both yoga therapist and client—there is no right or wrong way to perceive sensation. In a posture that lengthens part of a client's body, I might ask if the experience of length is soft or hard; diffuse or localized; rigid or fluid. If someone is in a posture that engages muscles, strengthening an area, I might ask how he experiences that sensation of muscular work: Does this feel strong or weak; Is the sensation diffuse or localized; Does it feel stable or unstable?

When a client is new to meditation in asana, I help them to find a posture that they perceive as safe, supportive, and restorative, as this inquiry takes some time. While people are learning to develop nonjudgmental observation, curiosity, and discrimination of sensation through the koshas I want them to feel safe, comfortable, and at ease—the qualities of sattva guna and a regulated body-mind. Chapter 11 continues this exploration with postures that the client finds challenging.

Practice 10.2 Asana Kosha Meditation

Consider starting with supportive postures (e.g., constructive rest, mountain brook, supported fish, supported bound angle, supported bridge; see Figures 9.2, 9.13, 9.14, 9.12, and 9.3). The posture needs to be one that can be comfortably sustained. The first time you do this reflective exercise, you may choose to meditate only on annamaya. During subsequent sessions, you might add one, two, or all of the other koshas, as tolerance allows.

Annamaya Reflection

- Where does this posture bring your attention? As you notice that sensation, what is its quality? Is it open or closed, heavy or light, bright or dark, hard or soft, fluid or rigid, diffuse or localized?

Pranamaya Reflection

- Does this sensation change with the phases of breath—during the inhale and exhale? If so, how? How does the breath affect this sensation? If you imagine breathing into this area, what do you notice?
- To explore more abstract ideas of energy, we can relate sensations to the gunas, prana vayus, colors, images, and so on. Does the sensation have a quality of calm or clarity, agitation or activity, groundedness or dullness? As you focus on this sensation, is there an image, quality, or word that wants to come in or be released? Does a color or image arise?

Manomaya Reflection

- As you continue to focus on this area of your body, maintaining the posture, are there thoughts or emotions that arise? If so, can you observe them and notice the qualities? Are they heavy or light, bright or dark, hard or soft, calm or agitated or dull?

Vijnanamaya Reflection

- Some descriptions of this kosha include beliefs. Are particular beliefs arising as you continue to hold this position? If so, can you observe them and notice their qualities?
- To reflect on the quality of discrimination, notice this capacity to observe sensations of the body and mind. Notice how these sensations arise, grow and move, shift and change, and fall away. Can you connect to the quality of the observer? How do you notice this? Is there a color, image, or shape? Are you behind the sensations, over them, around them?

Anandamaya Reflection

- As you observe these sensations, can you step back and notice the presence of qualities such as contentment or equanimity? Does an image, memory, word, or affirmation strengthen this sense of equanimity amidst the other sensations?

Clinical Example

"Jamal" had symptoms of anxiety and shoulder pain. We worked in supported fish to bring attention to the opening of the chest and shoulders. Jamal was comfortable in this posture and felt it helpful both for shoulder pain and for creating an experience of calm and clarity that supported inquiry.

- Annamaya: He felt the sensation as sharp, hard, rigid, and localized in the front of the chest and right shoulder.
- Pranamaya: The sensation in this area of the body created a feeling of stuckness and difficulty inhaling. The image that arose was of a brick wall, impenetrable and protective.
- Manomaya: Jamal perceived the emotion of fear behind the wall. It was circular, dark, and heavy.

- Vijnanamaya: The belief that arose was one of being unsure about the ability to let go of this fear. Jamal felt that it might not be OK to either voice or feel this fear. We worked with what it meant to observe these sensations. He could stand behind the wall and behind the dark, heavy circle that represented the fear.
- Anandamaya: Jamal was able to experience a feeling of equanimity with an image of his family, picturing them encircling these sensations along with him.

Jamal visualized each family member in the circle helping to take down the wall brick by brick. He felt supported, comforted, and contented as the wall came down and was able relax into the openness of the posture. Jamal's fear naturally dissipated as he felt this support.

In addition to inquiring into sensations while in postures, we can help people to explore how postures shift their experiences even afterward. Additional time in a restful position allows for reflection on physical sensation, energy level, breath quality, and thoughts and emotions. This opportunity to notice the effects of movement and posture can lead to significant insight and serve as a strong motivator for home practice.

Pranayama as Svadhyaya and Inquiry

What happens in our bodies as we breathe (movement of the lungs, respiratory diaphragm, etc.) can be subtle and difficult to sense, so I often use a visual aid to familiarize clients with the anatomy of respiration. Using a book or app, we look at images of the lungs, respiratory diaphragm, ribs, and pelvic floor and discuss how these structures move with inhalation and exhalation. This imagery can then be incorporated into visualizations during a pranayama-focused meditation such as Practice 10.3.

Practice 10.3 Pranayama Kosha Meditation

This meditation encourages recognition of the effects of the breath along the koshas.

Annamaya Reflection

- As you breathe, notice the movement of the ribs, abdomen, chest, pelvis and pelvic floor, shoulders, and arms—motions on the inhale

and exhale. Perhaps on inhalation gentle expansion occurs throughout the body—even through the arms, pelvis, and legs—allowing the breath to be received. You might also notice that the body settles back on exhalation with a gentle inward turn of the legs and arms. Are there parts of the body that move more easily or less easily through the breath cycle? Are there areas to which you feel more or less connected?
- Notice the sensation in the body during each part of the breath cycle. How does it change during inhalation, pause and transition, and exhalation? Where does sensation settle in the body with each part of the cycle? What is the quality of those sensations? Open or closed, heavy or light, bright or dark, fluid or rigid?

Pranamaya Reflection

- To explore the gunas and prana vayus, reflect on questions like the following. During the full cycle of breath—or during each stage—do you notice a sense of calm or clarity, agitation or activation, groundedness or dullness?
- How do you experience the inhale and receiving of the breath, the exhale and letting go of the breath, the pauses in between, and the overall fluidity of the breath? Which parts are easeful and comfortable, and which are uncomfortable or difficult?
- Do any images or colors arise during each phase of breath or through the full cycle?

Manomaya Reflection

- Notice any emotions or thoughts that arise during each phase of breath or through the breath cycle. Can you observe these thoughts and locate them in the body? What is their quality? Heavy or light, bright or dark, calm, agitated, or dull?

Vijnanamaya Reflection

- Are there beliefs that arise as you breathe? Notice the qualities of these beliefs.
- Notice the capacity to observe the physical sensations, movement of the breath, turnings of the mind—how all of these arise, grow, shift, and fall away. Just as the breath is fluid, so are the sensations of the body and mind.

> *Anandamaya Reflection*
>
> - Can you notice, alongside the breath and body-mind sensations, the qualities of steadfast equanimity or contentment present through each breath phase? Is there an image, memory, word, or affirmation that helps connect you to this equanimity and calm amidst all the other sensations of the body-mind?

Clinical Example

"Erikah" was experiencing pelvic pain and difficulty sleeping. We worked first in constructive rest and moved to supported bridge (see Figure 9.3) with a blanket underneath the pelvis. The torso angle created by this support allowed greater connection to the breath's movement because of the perception of resistance against gravity on the inhale and facilitation of relaxation of the respiratory structures as they moved with gravity on the exhale.

- Annamaya: Physically, Erikah's inhalation felt restricted, with less mobility in the pelvis and abdomen and more mobility in the shoulders and chest. The exhalation felt short and restricted. She experienced the rhythm between inhales and exhales as disjointed and often different from one breath to the next.
- Pranamaya: In energetic terms, the inhale felt calm and the exhale felt agitated and uncomfortable.
- Manomaya: Erikah's thoughts and emotions in this meditation centered on concern about allowing too much motion or relaxation to occur in the pelvis and abdomen—she felt that this might cause the pain to increase. Her worry felt heavy and dark in the lower abdomen and pelvis.
- Vijnanamaya: A belief arose that it was not OK to relax. Erikah perceived this idea as dark, heavy, and agitated in the lower abdomen and pelvis.
- Anandamaya: Erikah could experience feelings of equanimity when she brought the image of an ocean into her body.

From this image of the ocean, we could work with the breath matching the movement of the ocean. Erikah also used an affirmation of "I am safe" on the inhale with the image of waves coming onto a shore. She affirmed "I allow" on the exhale as the waves returned to the stillness and depths of the ocean. Gradually she was able to feel her body let go of resistance on the inhale and experience greater relaxation on the exhale with a more fluid breath. As Erikah found that she could safely experience physical relaxation, the worry and concern dissipated. She experienced her breath as light and expansive and felt both greater connection to, and capacity to relax in, her abdomen and pelvis.

More Meditations for Svadhyaya and Inquiry

In addition to the meditations above, I use others for cultivating svadhyaya, interoception and proprioception, and discriminative wisdom.

Prana Vayu Meditations

We might focus on the elemental forces of prana and apana vayu as starting points for inquiry and discriminative wisdom. (See Practice 5.1, p. 98 for a brief reflection on the prana vayus, and Practice 11.1, p. 243 for additions that develop greater body-mind resilience.)

> **Practice 10.4 Prana and Apana Vayu Meditation**
>
> Find a comfortable position and close your eyes if you like. Notice sensations both outside and inside your body. Notice sensations in the mind—emotions, thoughts, and beliefs. Without changing anything, simply notice.
>
> You might choose to next explore each vayu's energetics in turn, or to focus on one type of energy.
>
> *Prana Vayu*
>
> - Notice whether a particular quality would like to be received, supported, or manifested. This sense could come from the body (e.g., openness, groundedness), or from the mind (e.g., peace, gratitude, love, or an attribute like forgiveness). Ask the body and mind what wants to be brought in. Notice if an image or word arises, if movement wants to happen. If so, allow these. Play for a moment with images, words, or movement to see what happens when you permit this expression.

- This practice could take the form of anything from an image, such as an ocean or mountain, to movement, such as restorative or dynamic postures or a walk outside. Allow what wants to come into the system to do so.

Apana Vayu

- What needs to be released? Is there something to let go of so as to more fully receive the above intention of prana vayu—or any other intention that wants to be received? Are there tensions or places of disconnection in the body? Do thoughts, emotions, or beliefs resist this letting go or bringing in of an intention? What might need to happen to let go of these tensions or beliefs? Does an image, word, or movement arise to signify the resistance to receiving something different?
- You may notice resistance in the form of sadness, guilt, fear, confusion, or shame. Rather than delving into the cognition of what this means, can you experience these emotions in your body, in the present? Can you explore how you want to meet these sensations?
- An image of nurturing, comfort, or safety may arise. Let those images assist the apana vayu qualities in being seen, held, loved, or resolved. A position or movement may arise to provide comfort or kindness to meet this experience of apana vayu. Notice what is needed to let this body-mind resistance be seen and to allow yourself to experience the intention you want to bring in.

Integration

- Take a few moments to explore how to meet what wants to come in—prana vayu—and what needs to happen to release and let go—apana vayu.
- For example, openness that wants to come in may be resisted by fear. Experience the fear and ask what movement, image, or word is needed for resolution and to allow the openness in—maybe a restorative and comforting position, maybe an enlivening and strengthening one, or maybe a fluid and dynamic one. Let that happen.

Clinical Example

"Celia," who had low back pain, was in constructive rest (see Figure 9.2) during the meditation in Practice 10.4. She wanted to bring in the attribute of forgiveness during the prana vayu part of the meditation, but she was unable to connect to a way to facilitate that. We moved to the apana vayu part of the meditation, and Celia recognized that she wanted to let go of a feeling of anger, which she sensed as a hard, heated sensation with an agitated energy and a clenching throughout her body. This feeling was most pronounced in her pelvis and lower abdomen.

Celia explored these body-mind feelings to inquire into what was needed to let them go and bring in forgiveness. We explored supported forward folds, supported bound angle, bridge, gentle flowing postures with the breath (e.g., supine twists), seated sidebends, and modified sun salutes. The movement with breath with modified sun salutes and bridges connected Celia to an experience of fluidity and allowing, giving her an idea of how forgiveness might feel. We worked with breath-linked movement to strengthen her capacity for the experience of allowing, spaciousness, and nonjudgment. Eventually, Celia was able to return to constructive rest position and bring nonjudgmental expansiveness to the anger. Over time, the clenching and agitation began to dissipate. Celia found greater ease, relaxation, and an ability to let sensations, thoughts, and ideas move through. Her home practice continued this work.

Body Scan

Body scans develop nonjudgmental observation, discriminative wisdom, and interoceptive and proprioceptive skills. Below is just one example of the many ways to do a practice like this. Different traditions recommend starting with the head, feet, or mouth. I often start with the head and end at the feet to support grounding. However, for some people—particularly those with headaches or who have agitated minds—starting at the feet, far from the head, seems to work well.

> **Practice 10.5 Body Scan**
>
> Find a comfortable position in supine, sitting, or any yoga asana.
>
> - Take a moment to settle into this position. Your eyes can be open or closed, but soften your gaze if you choose to keep them open.

- Notice the breath and allow it to become soft and effortless.
- In each section of the body listed below, simply notice each area without doing or changing anything. (The latter invitation is particularly useful for emphasizing purely nonjudgmental observation.)
- Body scan:
  - Notice the outline of your whole body.
  - Bring your attention to the crown of your head, to your eyes, ears, jaw, throat, neck. Notice the whole face and neck.
  - Bring attention to your right shoulder, left shoulder, right arm and hand to the fingertips, left arm and hand to the fingertips. Notice both arms.
  - Notice the front of the chest, heart space, abdomen, sides of the torso, and back of the torso. Trace down each vertebrae of the spine, the muscles alongside your spine. Notice the pelvis—front, side, and back. Notice the whole torso and pelvis.
  - Notice the right hip, left hip, right thigh and knee to foot and toes, left thigh and knee to foot and toes. Notice both legs.
  - Notice the whole outline of your body again.
- Possible additions (see Practice 11.2, p. 245 for more detail):
  - To begin with the articulation of sensation, explore questions like the following for each part delineated above. Notice places that are connected/disconnected; open/closed; hard/soft; fluid/rigid; bright/dark; heavy/light. (Chapter 11 builds on this articulation of sensation for resilience and transformation of experience.)
  - To invite a certain intention into each area, explore what quality is needed or wanted: softness or relaxation, openness or spaciousness, vitality or energy, groundedness or stability. As you move through the body, would any word, phrase, image, breath, or color be helpful for inviting this intention to the area? Adding intention facilitates connection to the attributes of sattva guna, body-mind regulation, and grounding. Intention may also encourage the experiences you want to cultivate in the body. Intentions to direct to each part of the body include "may you find peace," "may you be filled with loving-kindness," "may you find ease," or "may you be filled with vitality."

Conclusion

From a foundation in sattva guna, body-mind regulation, and activation of the social engagement neural platform, yogic practices can be directed toward development of insight into the body-mind and behavioral habits that contribute to suffering. Through a biomedical or neurophysiological lens, this work includes building proprioceptive and interoceptive skills for improved recognition and identification of sensations in the body and mind. Through a yoga lens, we can develop discriminative wisdom based on the framework of samkhya and yoga provided in Chapters 3 and 4 (purusha/prakriti, gunas, buddhi/ahamkara/manas, kleshas, prana vayus). We can understand these insights through the koshas and biopsychosocial-spiritual models.

The practices in this chapter aim to foster healthy proprioception and interoception. In the realm of annamaya, we can support clients in identifying physical positions or movements that encourage qualities such as ease, strength, and stability. Cultivating a relationship to inner bodily sensation with a compassionate attitude of nonjudgmental observation promotes connection to oneself.

Recognizing subtle sensation, on the energetic level of pranamaya, is part of increasing sensitivity. Interoceptive skills are deepened through awareness of the effects of breath, movement, imagery, and meditation on one's energy, vitality, and physical and mental/emotional experience.

Further developing the skill of kind, compassionate observation of thoughts, emotions, and beliefs involves manomaya, the kosha of the mind, and emotion. The framework of yoga is particularly helpful for disentangling these different aspects of the "mind" and how they are reflected in the body, in relationships with the world, and in one's life. We can support clients in observing with "bare" awareness their thoughts, emotions, and beliefs as well as the effects of various practices on these aspects of mind.

Svadhyaya is an essential ethical principle for working with vijnanamaya. We can tap into the wisdom of this kosha through self-study, developing sensitivity to and accurate interpretation of body-mind experiences. In this vital stage of yoga's transformative work we learn to identify habitual patterns that perpetuate suffering as well as new relationships to the body-mind to alleviate suffering. The practices in this chapter therefore build the capacity for nonjudgmental observation and discrimination among physical sensations, psychological processes, and actions. Ultimately, clients begin to identify the gunas and how they show up in the body-mind, discern the different aspects of mind, notice subtle energy, and recognize how yogic practices affect the body-mind system.

Ethical practices are an important aspect of spiritual well-being—anandamaya, the realm of bliss or awe. The self-study of svadhyaya helps to develop the deep personal connectedness that is part of both spiritual and eudaimonic well-being. From this type of inquiry, we can realize other aspects of eudaimonic well-being including self-actualization, self-realization, personal authenticity, and meaning-making. As svadhyaya is combined with other virtues, we learn to relate to body-mind stimuli with kindness and compassion. Eventually we extend these lessons to changing our relationships to external stimuli such as interpersonal relationships and life circumstance to promote ever greater spiritual and eudaimonic well-being.

Notes

1. For more information on these ideas, resources include: Tsay, A., Allen, T. J., Proske, U., & Giummarra, M. J. (2015). Sensing the body in chronic pain: A review of psychophysical studies implicating altered body representation. *Neuroscience & Biobehavioral Reviews, 52*, 221–232; Craig, A. D. (2015). *How do you feel? An interoceptive moment with your neurobiological self.* Princeton, NJ: Princeton University Press; Farb, N., Daubenmier, J., Price, C. J., Gard, T., Kerr, C., Dunn, B. D., ... Mehling, W. E. (2015). Interoception, contemplative practice, and health. *Frontiers in Psychology, 6*, 763; Haase, L., Stewart, J. L., Youssef, B., May, A. C., Isakovic, S., Simmons, A. N., ... Paulus, M. P. (2016). When the brain does not adequately feel the body: Links between low resilience and interoception. *Biological Psychology, 113*, 37–45; Strigo, I. A., & Craig, A. D. (Bud). (2016). Interoception, homeostatic emotions and sympathovagal balance. *Philosophical Transactions of the Royal Society B: Biological Sciences, 371*(1708), 20160010. https://doi.org/10.1098/rstb.2016.0010; Pearson, N., Prosko, S., & Sullivan, M. (Eds.). (2019). *Yoga and science in pain care: Treating the person in pain.* London: Singing Dragon.
2. Farb et al., Interoception, contemplative practice, and health; Fiori, F., Aglioti, S. M., & David, N. (2017). Interactions between body and social awareness in yoga. *Journal of Alternative and Complementary Medicine, 23*(3), 227–233; Haase et al., When the brain does not adequately feel the body.
3. Many of the practices in this chapter are influenced by work and study with Julie Wilcox and Richard Miller.

Yogic Practices to Support Resilience and Transformation

11

This chapter highlights practices intended to transform habitual relationships with body-mind-environmental stimuli to support optimal well-being. These practices both evolve from and are supported by the body-mind regulation and sattvic qualities encouraged in Chapter 9 and the inquiry practices in Chapter 10.

The concept of resilience is key in shifting relationships to body-mind-environmental stimuli. Resilience, essential to effective transformation, includes the capacity to respond appropriately to stimuli and to move between states of activation and calm efficiently (see Chapters 7 and 8). I consider resilience to embody three key abilities, as outlined below.

Three Types of Resilience

1. Alternating Between Activation and Calm

I often begin working with resilience by introducing the idea of alternating between activating and calming practices. Activation does not always mean strengthening, nor does it always refer to the physical layer of experience. Likewise, deactivation does not always mean relaxing—it could also involve grounding, enlivening, or centering practices, on any layer of experience including the body, energy, or mind.

I invite clients to explore practices that create activation and calm in their own unique bodies, energy levels, thoughts, and emotions and to then move between the two states. Activating practices could include active or restorative postures; reflection on ethical principles that are difficult or uncomfortable to apply to oneself or one's life circumstances; difficult emotions or beliefs; or even breathing practices that arouse the person physiologically, energetically, or psychologically. Calming practices include any that bring a sense of confidence, inner strength, comfort, support, peace, or relaxation. They might take the form of either active or resting postures, reflection on various ethical principles, breathing practices, or meditations.

From a neurophysiological standpoint, we are moving between the neural platforms as discussed with polyvagal theory (Chapter 8), finding facility with coming back to social engagement after experiencing the other neural platforms. From a yogic standpoint, we are moving between the gunas and returning to sattva predominance.

2. Widening the Window of Tolerance

Alternating between arousal and calm can develop confidence and self-efficacy in the ability to manage one's relationship to body-mind-environmental stimuli. The capacity to be present with activation, without becoming overwhelmed, evolves from this practice. In terms of polyvagal theory, this type of resilience means ever greater bandwidth for states of safe mobilization and safe immobilization. In yoga, this resilience signifies increased ability to remain situated in sattva while noticing and experiencing greater fluctuations of rajas and tamas.

In other words, we can be present with and experience a wider spectrum of activation of the body and mind while still finding a degree of comfort and ease. For example, a client might perform a physically activating posture, like bridge, alongside a breathing technique or meditation that produces relative physical and mental ease. The intention is to increase the capacity to be with a broader spectrum of arousal while still accessing relatively calm physiological, positive psychological, and prosocial behavioral states.

As an example, a client who was initially suffering with social anxiety and claustrophobia, among other physical and mental conditions, demonstrates this regulation and resilience in action. During different therapeutic sessions, she had learned, for calming, both *sitali* ("cooling breath" with oral exhalation through a rolled tongue) and "grounding breath" (visualizing inhalations traveling up the body from the ground and exhalations traveling back down into the earth). When she later found herself in an extremely stressful situation—closed in a small room packed with strangers during a bomb threat—she was able to regulate her mental state and arrived at a combination of these two breathing practices. She inhaled "up" from the solid earth beneath her feet and exhaled a soothing stream from her mouth, again feeling rooted down. Although she'd never been taught to use these exercises together, by that time she had developed sufficient independence with these techniques to identify and execute a useful practice rather than falling into a habitual reaction, which might previously have been a panic attack or outright collapse. While many of those around her became visibly agitated and eventually angry, she was able to maintain regulation of her system and even take necessary actions immediately after the threat ended.

3. Transforming Relationships to Stimuli and Fluctuations

Yoga also teaches another approach to changing our relationships to stimuli. Once we realize our essential nature as awareness, we can experience these natural, inevitable fluctuations (of neural platforms, gunas, body-mind-environmental stimuli) with equanimity. Beyond building a greater capacity to observe stimuli, we can learn to embrace and welcome all experience as awareness, leading to eudaimonic well-being and steadfast contentment. (Although we may often conceptualize transformation as sweeping change, we must consider that transformation may more often consist of the subtle and incremental.)

A story in the Mahabharata has been helpful to me in understanding this facet of resilience. During the epic's central battle, the army opposing the Pandavas released the powerful Narayana weapon, which unleashed a torrent of fiery missiles and arrows. Many of the warriors in the Pandava army were decimated, and the harder they fought, the mightier the weapon became. Krishna told the stunned warriors that the only way to survive would be to cease fighting and lay down their arms: The more force and resistance the Narayana weapon meets, the more powerful it becomes. Everyone followed Krishna's directions except Bhima. Son of the wind god and the embodiment of will, Bhima refused to stop fighting. Instead, he rushed on, determined to conquer this weapon. Just as Krishna said, the Narayana met Bhima's ferocity by itself growing in strength. Krishna rushed to persuade Bhima, reassuring him that they would fight more intensely if that were indeed the way to defeat this weapon. Bhima finally listened, laying down his weapon and ceasing to fight. At that point, the Narayana passed over the army, dissipating and enabling the Pandavas to revive.

This story helps to describe an essential teaching of yoga. Sometimes deliberately altering sensations and experiences is beneficial in changing our relationship to stimuli of the body, mind, and environment. However, at other times this effort only makes the reactions more resistant to change. Rather than using greater intensity or strength, yoga teaches another approach to navigate these naturally arising fluctuations.

Just as the Narayana weapon loses its charge when resistance ceases, when we realize all experiences as part of awareness, we find the ability to meet stimuli differently. A capacity to allow stimuli to arise, rather than needing to change or manipulate them, enables an experience of steadfast contentment and eudaimonic well-being amidst the fluctuations of the body-mind-environment. It is important to emphasize that this teaching is not meant to foster unhealthy detachment or staying in dangerous or unhealthy situations. Rather, acceptance of what is present allows for an openness and responsiveness toward right action from which healthy physiological, positive psychological, and prosocial behavioral states emerge.

These final three chapters in this book can be understood as an evolution in one's practice. Yoga helps us to develop the ability to regulate the body-mind for greater safety and calm (Chapter 9), develop insight into patterns that perpetuate suffering (Chapter 10), and transform our relationship to stimuli for the cultivation of deep peace and equanimity (Chapter 11).

Yama and Niyama

Tapas, Svadhyaya, and Ishvara Pranidhana: Essential Principles for Resilience

Patanjali's Yoga Sutras list three constituents of active yoga practice: *tapas*, *ishvara pranidhana*, and *svadhyaya*. Engaging with these three ethical principles helps to "cultivate pure contemplation and attenuate the forces of corruption"[1] and provides insight for the development of resilience.

Tapas is the heat, friction, austerity, and disciplined practice needed for transformation and change. Through practice, we recognize habitual reactions that contribute to suffering, then apply fortitude, courage, and determination to transform these patterns so they instead support greater well-being. We must be willing to engage in the continued disciplined of steady practice for yoga's transformational processes to occur.

Ishvara pranidhana represents the capacity for allowing, and for being guided by, listening to, and trusting in a higher principle or power. The concept includes ideas of faith, devotion, and trust and reflects the practitioner's willingness to surrender to the highest expression of spirit or awareness.

Ishvara pranidhana helps us to develop the trust necessary to allow stimuli to arise, grow, shift, and fall away. This attribute balances the concept of tapas—the ability to stay with sensation and be present to what arises while trusting that the process will lead to what is needed for greater well-being.

Svadhyaya (self-study) provides the insight essential to navigate between the firm determination of tapas and the trustful allowing of ishvara pranidhana. The story of the Narayana weapon is a lesson on the importance of surrender or allowing; at other times, as in the Bhagavad Gita, the Mahabharata teaches the necessity of determination, engagement, and strong action for transformative change.

These three qualities provide the fortitude or determination (tapas), faith or trust (ishvara pranidhana), and self-reflection or insight (svadhyaya) needed for resilience. By cultivating these characteristics, we learn to stay present through levels of activation, when and how to return to states of calm before becoming overwhelmed, and to transform our relationships to sensations of the body, mind, and life.

Several practices in this book offer ways of contemplating tapas, ishvara pranidhana, and svadhyaya in relation to other concepts, including dharma (see Practice 2.1, p. 33), Aristotle's golden mean (see Practice 9.1, p. 186), and the yamas/niyamas (see Practice 10.1, p. 215).

Additional Ethical Principles

In addition to the three essential principles above, we could contemplate any yama or niyama for the development of resilience and for transformation. For example, someone may struggle with patience, forgiveness, or compassion, becoming uncomfortable or even agitated as they inquire into the meaning of these concepts in the context of their lives. Practices such as those mentioned above (2.1, 9.1, and 10.1) provide an opportunity for deep self-inquiry to transform habitual patterns from those that may be unhealthy or maladaptive to those that promote well-being.

Asana

Asana can be used with the intentions of alternating between states of activation and calm, widening the window of tolerance, and transforming relationships to stimuli by supporting an experience of steadfast contentment and eudaimonic well-being amidst the fluctuations of the body and mind.

Alternating Between Activation and Calm

Physiological resilience can be supported by alternating between postures that activate the systems of the body (e.g., sun salutations or standing postures that activate the cardiorespiratory, nervous, and musculoskeletal systems) and those that are more likely to result in calmer states (constructive rest or other restorative positions that support relaxation of these systems; see Figures 9.2–9.6, pp. 193–195). We can also help people identify postures or exercises that bring about mental activation or calm. Ideally, yoga therapy sessions support clients in self-exploration to identify postures that produce activated and calm states for them and to develop facility with moving between these states.

Clinical Example

"Maeve" was experiencing low back pain, migraines, depression, and fatigue. She often felt a sensation of weakness in her back with standing postures, as if her body could not support her; holding these poses created lower back discomfort or pain. Postures that created calm and safety and allowed Maeve to release tension included constructive rest and pigeon.

After we worked with inquiry practices (see, e.g., the asana kosha meditation in Practice 10.2, p. 221), Maeve was able to distinguish among different qualities of sensation. Rather than experiencing all sensation as pain, she was able to report when her back started to feel "fatigued" or "alert"—qualities she began to recognize as precipitating her pain. She would work on standing postures until she began to experience this alertness or fatigue, then come to constructive rest or pigeon until her back felt calm and rested. Over time, Maeve increased both the length of time she could stay in standing postures and the speed with which she could return to a relaxed physical and mental state.

Ultimately, Maeve developed confidence in her capacity to discern different qualities of sensation, listen to her body's needs, and identify practices that would help her improve function and ease any discomfort or pain.

Widening the Window of Tolerance

Once a foundational ability to move back and forth between activation and calm is established, I often work to support clients in co-activation of other neural platforms with social engagement and/or with strengthening sattva guna amidst rajas and tamas. In other words, we find relative calm physiological, positive psychological, and prosocial behavioral states alongside activation.

We might, for example, identify a physiologically challenging posture such as active bridge while encouraging a breath technique like long exhalation and meditation on calming imagery or loving-kindness. This work could also include postures that create charged thoughts or emotions. Here, too, the client would come into the posture while employing breath or meditation practices that promote relative physical ease and mental calm.

Our intention is to support people in finding relative calm, ease, or sattvic states as they experience inevitable body-mind stressors. Inquiries that widen the window of tolerance to stimuli are described in detail in the body scan and introspective asana of Practices 11.2 (p. 245) and 11.3 (p. 247), respectively.

Clinical Example

"Shui" originally came to me with abdominal and low back pain. After a few months of working together, these areas were relatively pain-free. Shui was able to function with more ease and had a home program that helped her to manage discomfort. She had reached a point where she wanted to increase her function even more but had concerns about building strength and endurance as this had created more pain for her in the past.

We decided to explore bridge because that pose had previously increased her pain but would also strengthen key musculature to support her back for increased function and activity. As Shui did this posture, we built on the inquiry practices from Chapter 10 (interoception, proprioception, and the asana kosha meditation from Practice 10.2, p. 221). She was able to notice fear and tension arising in her body as she held bridge and used attention to the breath as a way to remember to bring ease into the posture. She noticed her tendency to react to the fear—and to any sensation in her back or abdomen—by tightening her jaw, shoulders, and low back. In addition, Shui noticed that she was not engaging muscles, including her gluteals and quadriceps, that could help her in the posture. She practiced mindfully engaging these muscles in a way that helped her release tension in her jaw and low back. Shui's fear began to dissipate as she noticed that she could be present with sensation and mindfully create change to increase strength, comfort, and ease. This practice helped her to feel more confident in her ability to strengthen her body and increase her endurance so that she could return to full participation in life activities.

Transforming Relationships to Stimuli and Fluctuations

Actively engaging relative calm in the body and mind is one way of increasing the capacity to abide with various stimuli. However, yoga also teaches a way of transforming our relationship to stimuli as we realize both our essence and all stimuli of the body, mind, and life as awareness. Deep equanimity and contentment amidst fluctuating stimuli emerge. Rather than manipulating or changing sensation, we learn to allow and embrace it.

Clinical Example

"Sam," who had recently experienced a number of stressors in her professional and personal lives, was dealing with anger and hip and leg pain and numbness.

We began work with a body scan (Practice 11.2, p. 245). Later, in the introspective asana of Practice 11.3 (p. 247), she experienced the idea of equanimity first through the image of an animal, a bear. For her, the bear image provided feelings of safety, support, and inner strength, indicating to Sam that she was able to allow and handle whatever might arise.

Pigeon pose created the optimal amount of sensation in her hip and leg to explore physical sensations of pain and her experience of anger. Sam was able to hold the posture while cultivating safety and support using the imagery of the bear. She described how the sensations in her hip and leg moved into anger, which then changed to sadness and eventually fatigue. As she stayed with these body-mind sensations, she noticed that they continually shifted, changed, and even dissipated in strength. She found that she was able to sustain inner strength and equanimity as these other sensations moved through her experience.

As part of her home practice, any time she felt discomfort in her body she would either come into pigeon or close her eyes in any position. She was able to bring to mind the image of a bear and then experience safety, inner strength, and contentment amidst other sensations. Sam noticed sensations like discomfort, anger, sadness, and fatigue, and she also noticed that they dissipated and morphed into other sensations.

Ultimately, Sam found that whenever anger, stress, or pain arose she could be present to them. Rather than ignoring, resisting, or trying to change these sensations they became indicators for her to assess and explore what was needed in that moment. Sometimes she discovered insight into necessary action. Other times, she found that she simply needed to be present and allow the sensations to arise and dissipate. She developed healthier relationships to her body, mind, and life, feeling increasingly confident in her ability to participate in day-to-day activities and experiencing an improved sense of well-being.

Pranayama

Pranayama practices can also act as catalysts for the physiological/psychological activation and calm helpful in cultivating resilience. Specific exercises such as right-nostril and high-frequency breathing (e.g., the "cleansing" kriyas of kapalabhati and bhastrika) are described in yogic texts as heat-generating or energizing. Contemporary research has found that these practices facilitate heightened physiological states as measured by autonomic nervous system parameters, attentional processes, and motor responses.[2]

In addition to physiological activation, working with the breath can create psychological activation. For some, respiratory patterns "supposed" to be calming can actually be activating. For instance, although many texts and research describe alternate-nostril breath as calming, many clients I have worked with find it difficult and describe the practice with words like "suffocating" or "claustrophobic." Similarly, although diaphragmatic breath is often calming, it can also be activating: Attention to the abdominal area may be uncomfortable or disconcerting or prompt judgment, shame, anger, and so on. Exercises that include high-frequency breathing, like kapalabhati, are thought to produce uplifted states: Some clients feel more vibrant, expansive, energized, and happy, whereas others may feel agitation.

One client who was ordinarily able to use alternate-nostril breath to calm herself provides an example: During a stressful work situation, she felt too anxious to use alternate-nostril breath and instead found kapalabhati more helpful in creating calm, relaxed energy. When someone is acutely stressed, trying to immediately shift their systems to stillness or calm is often unsuccessful and may create more harm by trying to force an opposite effect. Instead, an activating breath such as kapalabhati may "meet the individual's energy where it is" and help foster a state of invigorated calm.

As with asana, I explore with clients which practices they find activating and which they find calming; we can use the latter as a stable platform on which to introduce the former. However, for clients who find calm or stillness to be more challenging and agitating, we might begin with a foundation of activation as the more comfortable state for that person. This approach is useful for those who have a habit of "powering through" difficulties and for whom states of activation are the norm, including people who have experienced trauma or are used to living with heightened stress. Regardless of which practices we begin with, the person is invited to explore their ability to navigate between calm and activation. The capacity to tolerate activation while maintaining relative calm builds, and ultimately they connect to eudaimonic well-being amidst the body-mind's fluctuations.

Clinical Example

"Aria's" case illustrates how we can work with all three aspects of resilience. With a history of eating disorder and current abdominal pain, diaphragmatic breathing was both physically difficult and emotionally activating for her. She reported difficulty and resistance in connecting to her abdomen; when she did bring her attention to this part of her body, she experienced anger and sorrow. Because Aria had a history of an eating disorder, I worked in conjunction with this client's psychologist.

A calming pranayama for her was simple breath awareness, which I taught as effortless, easeful breathing. She simply noticed her inhale and exhale without needing to do or change anything. The breath did not need to look or feel like anything or to occur in any particular pattern.

Aria connected well with the chakra model and was interested in this idea of subtle energy. She created a meditation practice on the third chakra—*manipura,* in the area of the solar plexus—and what it meant to her to experience strength, inner will, and self-confidence. The color green symbolized this experience for Aria, and she was able to allow this color to pervade her body to create an expansive strength. Supported fish pose also helped her to connect to the third chakra and this meditation.

Alternating Between Activation and Calm

Eventually, we returned to diaphragmatic breathing, moving between consciously mobilizing the abdomen with the breath (activation for her) and effortless breathing in supported fish (calm for her). Over time, Aria realized that she could return to the effortless breath at any moment without becoming overwhelmed by body-mind sensation.

Widening the Window of Tolerance

We then began to explore what it would be like to stay with the agitation of diaphragmatic breath while maintaining a meditative focus on the third chakra, green light, and feeling of inner confidence. Aria decided to connect this imagery to the movement of her abdomen in rhythm with the breath: On each inhale, she expanded the green light from the third chakra into her entire abdomen; on the exhale, she allowed the feeling of confidence to move through her whole body with the green light.

Aria reported being able to experience feelings of sorrow or anger in her abdomen alongside a sense of inner strength. She was able to compassionately observe these difficult sensations and envelop them in the green light, inner strength, and confidence. Over time, the sorrow and anger could be held within, nurtured by, and even become part of her sense of strength.

Transforming Relationships to Stimuli and Fluctuations

As we continued working together, Aria explored this idea of changing the relationship to sensations in her abdomen and to sorrow and anger. She worked with the concept of remaining situated in her experience of strength and confidence while allowing for the natural movement of emotions and sensation, including discomfort. She noticed how these phenomena shifted and moved to different areas of her body. She noticed that they would sometimes become really strong, then weaken and even disappear entirely. She realized that while sensations of discomfort, anger, and sorrow came and went, the sense of strength was steadfast. Aria's resistance to her discomfort and anger disappeared as she recognized that her unwavering sense of inner confidence could help her to safely navigate body-mind sensation.

Meditation

Meditation is a key yogic practice for cultivating resilience, as demonstrated by its incorporation throughout the practices for yama/niyama, asana, and pranayama above.

Meditations can also be focused with specific intentions for the three aspects of resilience. Those that foster calm or ease (e.g., affirmations, focus on the breath, mantra, visualization) can be used after an activating practice to create greater facility in moving between states of activation and calm. Meditations can help with maintaining relative calm in the body-mind *during* an activating practice to widen the tolerance to sensations of the body-mind. In addition to those given in the pranayama and asana sections above, examples in this book include meditations on dharma, purusha and prakriti, and the gunas (see Practices 2.2, p. 44; 3.1, p. 56; and 3.2, p. 65, respectively). Finally, meditations can lead to a transformation in relationship to sensation

Practices for Resilience and Transformation 243

as we realize our essential nature—and all fluctuating stimuli of the body, mind, and life—as awareness. Meditation expands the possibilities for steadfast contentment and eudaimonic well-being amidst these natural oscillations. Such practices include meditations on the prana vayus (see Practice 5.1, p. 98); for experiencing the body, mind, and environment as awareness (see Practice 5.2, p. 102); and on a story like that of the Khandava forest (see Practice 5.3, p. 103). Additional meditations for resilience include those in Practices 11.1 to 11.3.

Practice 11.1 Vayu Meditation: Focus on Samana, Udana, and Vyana

This practice follows from the prana and apana vayu meditation in Chapter 10 (see Practice 10.4, p. 226). The first part of this meditation, in the previous chapter, focuses on inquiring into the qualities needing to be received as attributes of prana vayu and the qualities needing to be released as attributes of apana vayu. This second half focuses on the qualities of integration (samana), articulation (udana), and fluid change (vyana) for greater resilience and transformation.

You may want to revisit the practices for prana and apana vayu. You might choose to next explore each vayu's energetics in turn, or to focus on one type of energy.

- Find a comfortable position and close your eyes or focus inward. Notice sensations outside your body and inside your body. Notice sensations in the mind—emotions, thoughts, beliefs. Without changing anything, simply notice.
- Reflect back on what wants to be brought into your experience—to be received by the body and mind as this quality of prana vayu. This can be an image, word, or felt sensation. Reflect also on what wants to be let go as this quality of apana vayu—perhaps physical tension, imagery, word(s), or felt sensation.

Samana Vayu

- Begin to integrate these two ideas of bringing in and letting go. What new image, word, physical sensation, or movement emerges to express these complementary experiences? What do you need to learn from this integration of prana and apana vayu to enable you to be with these qualities differently? What new experience is being called for from this integration of receiving and releasing—a platform from which the intention of prana vayu can be felt, apana vayu can be released, and a new experience can emerge?

For example, if you are bringing in compassion as a quality of prana vayu and tension or fear arises as a quality of apana vayu to resist that intention, what new experience could be cultivated in the body-energy-mind as a quality of samana vayu? Does a new understanding of compassion, tension, or fear need to emerge? What new experience—strength, confidence, allowing, patience, contentment—is being called for? What movement, image, or thought creates this new experience in the body?

Udana Vayu

- How would you express or articulate this new experience of integration, of samana vayu? What kinds of feelings are present in the body, and what experiences or images arise in the mind? Can you describe this so that it can become a new learned pattern, a new way of inhabiting the body-energy-mind (e.g., expansion, connection, presence, strength, attention to the back of the body)?

Vyana Vayu

- This vayu represents the embodiment of fluidity, dynamism, and change. What new ways of being in the body emerge? What kinds of movements or postures may reflect this change? What kinds of new beliefs are needed to allow this new way of being in the body, mind, or life? What thoughts and emotions would be part of this new way of meeting stimuli? Can you create a template of this experience in the body-energy-mind to help you remember this new perspective?

Integration

- Can you find a new energetic, physical, or mental/emotional pattern to embody what you learned from what you are bringing in (prana vayu), what you may be resisting (apana vayu), how you are integrating the experience (samana vayu), and how you are articulating it (udana vayu)? Does a new way of understanding and being with the body, mind, or life emerge (vyana vayu)?

Clinical Example

Recall the example of Celia from Chapter 10 (p. 228). Initially, her work focused on prana and apana vayus: She wanted to explore prana vayu by bringing in the attribute of forgiveness and apana vayu by letting go of anger, which she felt as a clenching, hardness, and agitation.

Celia found that she felt forgiveness as an allowing spaciousness of letting things move through. She was able to apply this idea to the clenching and agitation in her body for a greater sense of ease and relaxation. Over time, we built on this to work with changing her relationship to sensation and cultivating resilience by adding the qualities of samana, udana, and vyana vayu.

Celia explored what it would mean to experience her anger and tension differently. Rather than resisting these sensations, she considered what it would mean to welcome and allow them with confidence in her ability to navigate these difficult experiences. She reflected on how to embrace and build healthier and more accepting relationships with these sensations.

She determined that her new experience (samana vayu) would need to be strength and inner confidence alongside softness and loving-kindness. Celia articulated this sensation (udana vayu) in two ways. First, she found that she could rest into her back body as a line of support from the soles of her feet to the crown of her head. From this sensation, she could access softness, openness, and receptivity in her front body—more specifically from the forehead to the heart space. Celia used standing postures with this reflection on strength in the back and openness in the heart to reinforce her experience. Over time, she developed a sense of trust in the back body providing inner strength and had the confidence to be open and able to respond appropriately to sensations of the body, mind, and life (vyana vayu). Celia found a capacity to both feel more open in her relationships and to create boundaries when necessary. She was able to listen to and respect her own needs and to support herself and those around her (vyana vayu).

> ### Practice 11.2 Body Scan: Focus on Resilience
>
> This practice builds on the body scan in Practice 10.5 (p. 228), in which we simply notice sensations. These example additions facilitate aspects of resilience and transformational change.
>
> - To explore flexible attention, notice sensations, and their opposites, in the body. Move your attention back and forth between

feeling these opposite sensations (e.g., areas of connection/disconnection, hardness/softness). You might also practice noticing both activating sensations and calming sensations in the body and move attention between them. It might be helpful to use an image or word to foster a calm experience if one is not found in the body.
- To expand the ability to be present with activation, notice a sensation in the body, a way of breathing, an image, word, or affirmation that brings a sense of calm. Rather than moving back and forth between activation and calm, practice holding the experience of calm in your attention while noticing sensations of activation.
- The following example exercises to transform relationships to stimuli invite the exploration of physical sensation from a perspective of curiosity and inquiry. The intention is to learn a new way of relating and reacting to sensation. Rather than judging, resisting, or manipulating sensations, we can compassionately explore them from a perspective of spacious allowing, welcoming, and openness.

  Notice any part of the body that has a distinct feeling (painful, uncomfortable, empty, full), and find a part that embodies the opposite. Explore what each area might have to teach the other.
  - What does this place of connection/comfort/ease have to teach places of disconnection/discomfort/unease/pain?
  - Can you bring this connection/comfort/ease to places of disconnection/discomfort/unease/pain?
  - To avoid judging which area is good or bad, better or worse, I sometimes ask more generally which place has something to teach the other. Does the discomfort, pain, or disconnection have something to teach the comfort, ease, or connection or vice versa?

    For example, one client felt she needed to bring the heaviness of one shoulder to the lightness of the other to create grounding and stability. Another found that a withered, atrophied leg needed to be filled by the fullness of the other leg.
  - If you cannot locate an opposite in your body, is there an image or felt sense of what it would be like to have no pain or no discomfort? You might also recall a time when you felt no pain or discomfort. Where and how do you notice that memory in your body?

    For example, a client with chronic leg and hip pain who was no longer able to work had very limited ability to be on his feet. He remembered what it was like to go waterskiing—the fluidity of his body moving, the sense of spaciousness and dynamism. He could visualize this in detail and feel a sense of fluidity in his body. Over time, he was able to bring this experience into his pain and to relax and feel greater ease around sensations of discomfort.

These practices encourage us to change our judgment toward our bodies by inquiring into healthier relationships to those areas. iRest Yoga Nidra is an excellent resource to support these transformations. The iRest Institute provides a framework and training from skilled practitioners on improving regulation, interoception and discernment, and resilience (see irest.us).

Practice 11.3 Bringing It All Together: Introspective Asana

This practice integrates techniques I learned from my mentor and teacher Julie Wilcox and with Richard Miller and the iRest Institute.

Encouraging Sattva Guna and Body-Mind Regulation

- Start in any comfortable, restful position. Work with a centering practice to help activate the parasympathetic nervous system and cultivate sattva. This might include a pranayama practice like longer exhales or a release of effort in breathing; setting an intention such as compassion for whatever arises; or bringing to mind an image or word that creates a sense of ease or peace. Encourage the capacity to nonjudgmentally observe sensations of the body-mind-environment.
- Set an intention. What do you want to cultivate or experience? Maybe let this become an affirmation (e.g., "I am filled with peace," "I am grounded and safe").
- Next, develop the experience of support, safety, inner wisdom, inner guidance, or peace. Consider all of these phrases and anything else that comes to mind to explore what resonates with you. The intention is for this experience to become a tangible one of safety and calm, which could arise from an image, memory, word, or felt sense. Can you locate this inner wisdom or support in your body? What are its qualities—color, appearance, feelings like

expansiveness or openness? Here we begin to learn what it means to connect to a safe place of inner support and wisdom. We will return to this experience throughout the practice to work with regulation, resilience, and transformational change.

One client reported a wide-open eye in her abdomen, looking around and almost hypervigilant. To soothe this feeling, she brought in the image of how when she pets her dogs their eyes begin to close. She pictured this eye being calmed in the same way. We were able to bring this image and feeling of her dogs supporting her and being soothed into experiences of activation and challenge.

Another person described an image of a lake encircled by hills and trees. When she sat on the banks of the lake, she felt the presence of a wise teacher and guide. Whenever discomfort or activation arose, she could rest on the lakeshore either in silence with this presence or asking for specific guidance.

Other clients have worked with a color that filled the body or with a phrase (e.g., "I am safe," "I can trust in the wisdom of this moment").

The above three steps might happen during a single session or over the course of several months, but they should be done before moving on.

Developing Interoceptive Skills and Discriminative Wisdom

Create the dialogue to explore sensations in the body. Like the practices in Chapter 10, this step involves developing curiosity and nonjudgmental observation of sensation. Questions to explore include:

- Where is your attention drawn in your body? Is there anything you are curious about in your body right now?
- What do you notice? How do you notice sensations, or how would you describe them in terms of textures, shapes, or colors? Are the sensations hard/soft, open/closed, fluid/rigid, bright/dark?
    - If thoughts or emotions arise, where or how do these show up in your body right now?
    - If articulating sensation is difficult, you might do a body scan. As you go through the different parts of the body, what do you notice? Places of tension, relaxation, heaviness, lightness, strength, weakness? You might also alternate between contracting and relaxing muscles to connect to physical sensation.

Building Resilience

- Is there a posture your body or mind wants to explore? (Alternatively, I might suggest a posture based on an assessment. Often, when I first work with someone I make the choice, but as the client develops proficiency in their practice and inner awareness they usually begin to choose which postures to explore.)
- Once in the posture, explore the sensations of it. Here we are building resilience by widening the spectrum of circumstance in which safe mobilization/safe immobilization is possible, or sattva can coexist with rajas/tamas. We are also encouraging flexibility by exploring the capacity to realize awareness and allow the fluctuations of the body-mind to move. Possible inquiries into sensations and in the postures include those suggested in Practice 11.2 and the following:
  - What sensations do you notice in this posture? How would you describe them? In shape, image, color? Do emotions, thoughts, or feelings arise?
  - What does this posture provide the opportunity to explore? A kind of connection to the body, a way of feeling or of understanding yourself? Maybe an experience of openness, strength, confidence, vitality, or ease? How can this posture serve you? Bring in this experience with any kind of breathing pattern, intention, image, word, or perhaps a different posture.
  - Can you allow spaciousness around the sensation? Can you stay with the sensations that arise and move, exploring what happens as you allow sensation to be present and to shift?
  - Does any emotion or thought arise from this sensation or posture? Where is this in the body? What is its shape, texture, color, or image? Is there something this emotion or thought needs? A different posture or an affirmation?
  - Can you notice the sensations of the body-mind and connect to inner wisdom, safety, or contentment? Be present to both this equanimity and to the body-mind's arisings.
  - How would you move from a place of support, comfort, or safety? From original intention and inner guidance?
- You might explore two to five postures with these kinds of questions and reflections.

> *Integration*
>
> - As an ending reflection, consider what arose and what was meaningful. What was interesting to you? What did you see or understand about the experience? What was meaningful to you?
> - What would serve as a useful longer-term practice? This might be a few of the postures, an image, or an affirmation.

Clinical Example

"Kevin" had upper back and neck pain. He wanted to work with symptoms of anxiety as well as stress and grief, which we explored through the introspective asana outlined in Practice 11.3.

To help foster a parasympathetic response, we began with constructive rest and lengthening the exhale as these practices were calming to him. I guided Kevin through a body scan, encouraging him to bring relaxation to each place.

Kevin wanted to find both comfort and a sense of inner confidence through this practice. He reported feeling this intention as a resting into the back body and allowing the waves of breath. With each inhale he used the mantra "I am," and with each exhale "I allow."

To find inner wisdom and support, Kevin thought of a mountain cabin, feeling the warmth of a fire and the open groundedness of nature. He experienced these sensations in his abdomen and was able to expand the warmth and openness into the rest of the body from there.

When asked where his attention was drawn, Kevin reported the neck, throat, and upper chest. The sensations there were dark, heavy, and fatiguing, and a feeling of being overwhelmed. Emotions included sadness and worry. We went back and forth between the inner wisdom of the mountain cabin and this experience of the throat. He was able to spend time in each place and to feel the safety in the abdomen even while experiencing the unpleasant sensations at the throat.

Asking the safety of the mountain cabin what might be helpful prompted the answer of a movement to open the chest and front of the shoulders, so we explored supported fish. Kevin noticed that the dark heaviness of his throat could be experienced with more spaciousness, so he explored his comfort with opening into this area. He allowed each inhale to fill the heart space to allow for a sense of motion, fluidity, and spaciousness to enter. In supported fish, Kevin could sense the heaviness, darkness, and overwhelm of the throat begin to move into the abdomen, into the cabin's space of safety. He was able to allow that mixing to happen. With the inhale he brought space and a sense of lightness to the throat and with the exhale invited sensation to be recognized and felt in the abdomen.

We explored what wanted to happen next with this feeling in the abdomen. He felt the darkness and heaviness held in healing, support, and safety. Because Kevin wanted some movement to increase the sensation's fluidity, we explored moving twists in rhythm with the breath. He was able to feel how the heaviness could become dynamic. He learned that he could feel grief, worry, and concern alongside ease, dynamism, fluidity, and openness. He sensed the confidence of being with strong sensation without overwhelm. We began to explore bringing the feeling of safety of the mountain home to this space.

At the conclusion of the practice, Kevin returned to constructive rest. He allowed a few breaths and noticed whether any areas needed to be relaxed.

Kevin found it meaningful to know that he had a capacity for safety in his body. The cabin in his belly became a safe refuge and meditation. He came away feeling that he had the confidence to be with strong mental and physical sensation and could work with them in such a way as to bring comfort and ease. Supported fish pose and moving twists became a home practice with a mantra of inhaling "I am" and exhaling "I allow."

Conclusion

The therapeutic yoga framework enables clients to understand the personal body, energy, and mind and how the relationship to oneself can either support or diminish well-being. Yogic practices can help people learn skills for body-mind regulation, interoception and discernment of sensation, and transformative resilience. Yoga therapists may take into account medical diagnoses, but these are not the driving force for the application of yogic practices. Rather, yoga focuses on helping us to explore the patterns of relating to the body, mind, and life that contribute to suffering. Yoga therapists then support clients in a process of change to facilitate greater physical, mental, social, and spiritual well-being.

A Case of Fibromyalgia

"Grace" had been diagnosed with fibromyalgia. She was experiencing generalized body pain, especially in the low back, hips, and shoulders, and dealing with both fatigue and difficulty sleeping.

We focused first on body-mind regulation for greater calm, ease, and relaxation. For several months, Grace and I explored yogic practices that would facilitate this ease as well as compassionate observation and loving-kindness toward herself.

We then worked on developing proprioceptive and interoceptive awareness. Grace learned to recognize and articulate sensation in a nonjudgmental, open manner. Because of her experience of pain and diagnosis of fibromyalgia, we focused on finding ways to normalize and create safe, healthy relationships to sensation. We discussed what compassion and loving-kindness meant and how Grace could begin to see sensations as guides or messengers for an improved relationship with her body, mind, and life.

Once Grace felt confident in returning to states of calm and in her ability to articulate sensations and recognize when they might become overwhelming, she started the resilience practices. We explored how she could experience the sensations of her body and mind alongside loving-kindness, contentment, and equanimity. Ultimately, Grace was able to recognize sensations within the body-mind, notice how life situations affected these sensations, and respond in ways that supported her well-being. Sometimes she found she needed to do practices for relaxation; at other times movement, walking in nature, or going out with friends was more helpful.

Grace learned how to navigate both her body-mind sensations and life circumstances in a positive manner to experience greater equanimity, contentment, and well-being. She changed the way she perceived herself, shifting from "someone with chronic pain with a few good days" to "someone who was enjoying her life and had a day here or there where she needed more rest or experienced some pain." Grace's pain no longer controlled her life, and she had tools to work with whatever arose while experiencing a deep contentment in herself and her relationships.

A Case of MS and Depression

With a diagnosis of multiple sclerosis, "Lucy" experienced fluctuating symptoms: Some days she had lots of vitality, energy, and clear-mindedness, and other days brought extreme fatigue and difficulty with physical and mental functions. This inconsistency in Lucy's capacity and energy left her feeling frustrated and unsure of what to expect from one day to the next. She wanted to build her endurance to participate in life activities and to explore patience in and acceptance of the natural variations that might occur in her daily physical, mental, and energetic levels.

As with Grace, we first spent a few months finding the practices Lucy needed to find a relaxed body and a calm, peaceful mind. We next worked on interoceptive and proprioceptive skills to support improved attention to body sensation. Lucy's physical practices emphasized recognizing physical, energetic, and mental cues to promote increased stability and strength while tuning into signals of fatigue. She learned to alternate practices of activation with rest to avoid overworking. She also learned to build endurance by staying present with activation, acknowledging sensations of the body-mind, and honoring cues to slow down.

Inquiry practices focused on exploring concepts like support, strength, and patience. Lucy learned to identify these ideas in how she related to her body, mind, and life actions. Over time, she developed the capacity for compassionate understanding and kind regard toward herself as she experienced greater contentment. Lucy was able to find ways to participate in daily activities as she wanted and to establish healthy boundaries that enabled her to acknowledge fatigue with compassion and kindness.

Notes

1. Miller, B. S. (1996). *Yoga: Discipline of freedom: The yoga sutra attributed to Patanjali*, p. 44. Berkeley, CA: University of California Press.
2. Telles, S., & Naveen, K. V. (2008). Voluntary breath regulation in yoga: Its relevance and physiological effects. *Biofeedback, 36*(2), 70–73; Raghuraj, P., & Telles, S. (2008). Immediate effect of specific nostril manipulating yoga breathing practices on autonomic and respiratory variables. *Applied Psychophysiology and Biofeedback, 33*(2), 65–75; Shannahoff-Khalsa, D. S., & Kennedy, B. (1993). The effects of unilateral forced nostril breathing on the heart. *International Journal of Neuroscience, 73*(1–2), 47–60; Telles, S., Nagarathna, R., & Nagendra, H. R. (1994). Breathing through a particular nostril can alter metabolism and autonomic activities. *Indian Journal of Physiology and Pharmacology, 38*, 133–137; Telles, S., Nagarathna, R., & Nagendra, H. R. (1996). Physiological measures of right nostril breathing. *Journal of Alternative and Complementary Medicine, 2*(4), 479–484; Bhavanani, A. B., Ramanathan, M., Balaji, R., & Pushpa, D. (2014). Differential effects of uninostril and alternate nostril pranayamas on cardiovascular parameters and reaction time. *International Journal of Yoga, 7*(1), 60. Telles, S., Singh, N., & Balkrishna, A. (2011). Heart rate variability changes during high frequency yoga breathing and breath awareness. *BioPsychoSocial Medicine, 5*(1), 4; Brown, R. P., & Gerbarg, P. L. (2005). *Sudarshan kriya* yogic breathing in the treatment of stress, anxiety, and depression: Part I—Neurophysiologic model. *Journal of Alternative & Complementary Medicine, 11*(1), 189–201.

Final Thoughts

Yoga therapy provides an important and unique perspective to support biopsychosocial-spiritual health and well-being. When the practices are situated within yoga therapy's foundational framework, they enhance systemic body-mind regulation, provide insight into the causes of suffering, improve resilience, and promote healthy, adaptive relationships with the circumstances of one's body, mind, and life. These effects illuminate yoga therapy's wide-ranging applications across client populations. Growing recognition of the influence of spiritual and eudaimonic well-being on biopsychosocial health further supports the significance of yoga's foundational wisdom and its application in therapeutic contexts. A challenge for the yoga therapist is to bridge the ancient wisdom of yoga with scientific understanding to ensure that the teachings and practices are accessible to both clients and other healthcare practitioners. We must therefore deeply understand for ourselves yoga's foundational teachings. A strong grasp of yoga therapy's explanatory model will likewise enable synergistic application of the practices to meet individual client needs. We need to cultivate the ability to readily articulate a shared language that will be well-received in multiple contexts and by different populations. This work will include exploration of other relevant philosophies and the language of neurophysiology and biomedicine.

As yoga therapy continues to grow and integrate into different healthcare settings, making its practices accessible while retaining their essence is imperative. Ultimately, evolving to reach a multitude of clients spanning different cultures, age groups, genders, and circumstances will ensure the practices' continued relevance.

Index

Page numbers in **bold** denote tables, those in *italics* denote figures.

abinivesha 82–3
action capacities *see* karmendriyas
adharma 105
affirmation practice 208–9
ahamkara 69, 71–2, 73, 74, 75–6, 84, 90, 95, 114
ahimsa 33, 185, 187
allostasis 135–6
allostatic load 136, 137, 138, 139, 142
alternate-nostril breathing 139, 206–7, 240
anandamaya kosha 89, 90, 93–4, **93**, 114–15, 128, 129
anandamaya reflection 222, 223, 225
Anderson, Sandra 95
annamaya kosha 88, 89, *89*, 91–2, *91*, 114, 127–8, 129
annamaya reflection 221, 222, 223–4, 225
ANS *see* autonomic nervous system (ANS)
anxiety 129
apana vayu 96, **96**, 171
apana vayu meditation 98, 227, 228, 243, 245
aparigraha 187
Aristotle 24, 36–7, 41, 42, 184
Arjuna 17, 18–19, 22, 31, 35, 38, 40, 41–2, 62, 63–4, 86–7, 107–8, 151
asana 15, 125–7, 139, *160*, 172–4; benefits of 172–4; for body-mind regulation 164, 188–96, 191–3, 193–201, 247–8; for discriminative wisdom 217–23; for interoceptive and proprioceptive skills 173, 217–23, 248; introspective 247–51; for resilience and transformation 236–40, 249; for sattva guna 164, 188–96, 191–2, 193–201, 247–8

asana kosha meditation 220–3
asana postures: bird dog *203*; bound-angle legs up the wall *198*; constructive rest *193*; figure-four legs up the wall *197*; half locust *202*; legs up the wall *197*; low lunge *196*; mountain brook *199*; plank *203*; single-leg standing *201*; starfish *195*; supine abdominal engagement *201*; supported bound angle *198*; supported bridge *194*; supported fish *199*; supported incline rest *194*; supported sidelying *195*; supported single-leg bridge *196*; supported twist *200*
asmita 81
asteya 187
attraction *see* raga
autonomic nervous system (ANS) 139, 143–8, *145*; definition 136–7; dysregulation 129, 147–8; polyvagal theory 144, 148, 149–53, 161, 162–3, **163**, *168*; pranayama and 171, 240
aversion *see* dvesha
avidya 80
awareness 20–7

Benson, Herbert 138
Bhagavad Gita *see* Mahabharata and Bhagavad Gita
Bhavanani, Ananda Balayogi 36, 133
Bhima 17, 31, 234
Bhishma 35, 61, 74, 75
bhramari breathing 206
bhutas 69, 74
biomedical model 18, 113, 132

Index

biopsychosocial-spiritual (BPSS) model 113; *see also* domains of health and well-being; psychophysiological perspectives
Blashki, Leigh 59
The Blind and Lame metaphor 52–3
bliss sheath *see* anandamaya kosha
body scans 33, 195, 209, 220, 228–9, 245–7
body-mind regulation: asana for 164, 188–96, 191–3, 193–201, 247–8; meditation practices for 164, 207–11; neurophysiological perspectives 137–42, 161; pranayama for 164, 204–7; psychophysiological perspectives 162–4, **163**; yamas and niyamas for 183–8, *184*; yoga therapy framework for 167–9; yogic perspectives 162–4, **163**; *see also* autonomic nervous system (ANS)
body-mind-environment (BME): constituents of prakriti 68–76, *69*, **70**, 78–9, 83–4; gunas in 59–64, 70–1, **70**, 72, 73, 75; from habitual response to insight 93–4, *93*; kleshas 80–3, *160*, 161; lived and habitual bodies 77–80, 84; meditation practices 101–4; phenomenology 76–80
bottom-up neurocognitive processes 139–42
brahmacharya 187
breathing practices *see* pranayama
Brihadaranyaka Upanishad 23, 79–80
buddhi 69–71, *69*, **70**, 73, 74, 75–6, 78–9, 83–4, 90, 95
buddhindriyas 69, 72–3, 74, 84

chakras 99, 101, 105, 106, 107
change, fear of 82–3
chariot metaphor 78
compassion meditation 138, 164, 175
connectedness 115, 117–18, *118*, 120, 125, 164
contentment *see* santosha
courage 184
cyclic meditation 167

The Dancer and the Dance metaphor 54–5
death, fear of 82–3
death-feigning response 151
defensive immobilization neural platform 151, 153, 162, *163*, **163**, 165, 167
defensive mobilization neural platform 151, 152, 162, *163*, **163**, 165, 167
depression 129, 252–3
dharana 174
dharma 30–47, 115; in action 39–40; buddhi and 70, **70**; definitions of 32; engagement with life and 37–8, 41–2; as guide to right action 32–6; personal expression of 34–6, 40–1; practices 33–4, 44–5; virtues and 32–6, 37; in yoga therapy 42–6, 47
dhyana 174

diaphragmatic breathing 204–5, 240, 241–2
discriminative wisdom 6, 52, 58, 90, 125, 127, *145*, 161; asana for 217–23; meditation practices for 220–9; pranayama for 223–6; yamas and niyamas for 214–17; *see also* buddhi
domains of health and well-being 114–22; eudaimonic well-being and 117–22, *118*, *119*; influence on health and well-being 116–17; and koshas 114–16, 127–9
Doniger, Wendy 31–2
dorsal motor nucleus 148, 149, 151, 153
dorsal vagal complex **163**, 168
dvesha 81–3

egoism 81
engagement with life 37–8, 41–2, 53
entextualization 100–1
ethical inquiry 43–4, 120–1, 125, 126, 127, 164; *see also* virtues; yamas and niyamas
eudaimonic well-being 24–5, 36–7, 40, 41, 161; engagement with life and 37–8, 41–2; health effects of 24–5, 122–3; meditation practice 210–11; practices 124, 210–11; spiritual domain of health and 117–22, *118*, *119*; in yoga therapy 25–7, 42–6, 47
existential connectedness 115, 117–18, *118*, 120, 125, 164
explanatory framework for yoga therapy 124–7, *126*; psychophysiological perspectives 159–66, *160*, **163**; yogic perspectives 159–66, *160*, **163**; *see also* domains of health and well-being; neurophysiological perspectives
exteroception 73, 144, *145*, 146–7, 150

fibromyalgia 251–2
fight-flight-freeze response 92, 129, 137
Finlayson, Diane 90, 92
Flood, Gavin 100–1
focused attention meditation 174–5
Frankl, Viktor 25, 40, 41, 42, 53, 121

gene expression 24–5
generosity 184
golden mean 184–6, *184*
granthis 99, 101, 105, 106, 107
gross elements 69, 74
gunas 57–66, *160*, 161; in body, mind, and environment 59–64, 70–1, **70**, 72, 73, 75; buddhi and 70–1, **70**, 73, 78–9, 83–4; definitions of 57–9; meditation practices for 65–6, 164, 207–11; neural platforms and 162–9, **163**, 168

habitual body 78–80, 84
hatha yoga 100

Index

Hatha Yoga Pradipika 170, 172
health: eudaimonic well-being and 24–5, 122–3; *see also* domains of health and well-being
heart rate variability (HRV) 139, 140–1, 150
hedonic happiness 24, 25–7, 60, 123
homeostasis 135, 136, 137, 147
humility 184
hypothalamic-pituitary-adrenal (HPA) axis 136, 137

identity 42–4, 52, 75–6, 78, 81–3, 106
ignorance 80
individuality *see* ahamkara
interoception 145–7, *145*, 148–9, 150, 161, 164
interoceptive skills: asana for 173, 217–23, 248; meditation practices for 220–9; pranayama for 223–6; yamas and niyamas for 214–17
introspective asana 247–51
iRest Institute 247
ishvara pranidhana 188, 235–6

Janda, Vladimir 191

karmendriyas 69, 72–3, 74, 84
Katha Upanishad 22, 25, 78
Khandava Forest 86–7, 104–8
kleshas 80–3, *160*, 161
Kornfield, Jack 207
kosha meditation: asana 220–3; pranayama 223–6
koshas 88–99, *89*, 100, 113, *160*, 161; anandamaya 89, 90, 93–4, *93*, 114–15, 128, 129; annamaya 88, *89*, 89, 91–2, *91*, 114, 127–8, 129; and domains of health and well-being 114–16, 127–9; manomaya 89, 90, 91–2, *91*, 114, 128, 129; pranamaya 88–9, *89*, 91–9, *91*, 114, 127–8, 129, 161; vijnanamaya 89, 90, 93–4, *93*, 114–15, 128, 129
Krishna 18–19, 22, 35, 38, 40, 41–2, 62, 63–4, 86–7, 107–8, 234

language, individualized shared 21–4
life experience *see* engagement with life
lived body 77–8, 84
loneliness 116–17, 128, 129
loving-kindness meditation 164, 175, 207–8

Mahabharata and Bhagavad Gita 5–6, 16–19, 22, 26, 151, 183; dharma 30–2, 34–6, 37–8, 39, 40–2; gunas 58, 59, 60, 61–2, 63–4; Khandava Forest story 86–7, 104–8; lived body 78; Narayana weapon story 234–5, 236; prakriti 51, 74, 75; prana vayus 95; purusha 50; resilience 166, 234–5, 236;

samkhya and yoga 49–50; yamas and niyamas 170
Mallinson, James 172
manas 69, 72, 73, 74, 75–6, 84, 90, 95, 114
manomaya kosha 89, 90, 91–2, *91*, 114, 128, 129
manomaya reflection 222, 224, 225
mantra meditation 175, 176, 208–9
meaning and purpose 24–5, 36, 37, 40–2, 115, 117, 119–20, 125, 127; engagement with life and 41–2, 53; one's own specific 40–1; in yoga therapy 25–7, 42–6, 47
meditation practices 15, 19–20, 28, 99, *160*, 174–6; affirmation 208–9; aspects of mind 75–6; benefits of 175–6; body scans 33, 195, 209, 220, 228–9, 245–7; for body-mind regulation 164, 207–11; body-mind-environment as awareness 101–4; cyclic 167; dharma meditation walk 44–5; for discriminative wisdom 220–9; eudaimonic well-being 210–11; for gunas 65–6, 164, 207–11; for interoceptive and proprioceptive skills 220–9; on Khandava Forest 108; loving-kindness 164, 175, 207–8; mantra 175, 176, 208–9; prana vayus 98, 226–8, 243–5; on purusha and prakriti 56–7; for resilience and transformation 242–7; for sattva guna 65–6, 164, 207–11
mental sheath *see* manomaya kosha
Merleau-Ponty, Maurice 77, 79
Miller, Richard 15, 32, 95, 99–100, 101, 165, 247
multiple sclerosis 252–3
Mundaka Upanishad 25–6
muscular inhibition 192
musculoskeletal balance 94, 173, 191–3, **193**

nadi shodhana 206
nadis 98–9, 101
Nakula 30, 31, 34
Narayana weapon 234–5, 236
neural platforms 144, 149–53, 161; gunas and 162–9, **163**, 168
neuroception 144, *145*, 148–9, 150, 151, 152
neurocognitive processes: bottom-up 139–42; top-down 138–9, 142
neurophysiological perspectives: regulation and resilience 137–42, 161; salutogenesis 132–6, *133*; *see also* autonomic nervous system (ANS)
niyamas *see* yamas and niyamas
nondual awareness practices 175
nonharming *see* ahimsa
nucleus ambiguus 148, 149, 150, 153

objective social isolation 116
open monitoring meditation 175

Pandavas: Arjuna 17, 18–19, 22, 31, 35, 38, 40, 41–2, 62, 63–4, 86–7, 107–8, 151; Bhima 17, 31, 234; Nakula 30, 31, 34; Yudhisthira 17, 30–1, 34–5, 41, 61, 74, 75
parasympathetic nervous system (PNS) 138, 139, 140–1, 143, 150, 162, 164, 168–9; asana and 173, 191; definition 137; meditation and 175; polyvagal theory 152–3; pranayama and 171, 204, 205, 206
Patanjali *see* Yoga Sutras of Patanjali
pathogenesis 132–3, **133**, 134
patience 185
Paul, Tina 185
perceived social isolation 116–17, 128, 129
phenomenology 76–80
physical domain of health 114, 127–8, 129
physical exercises *see* asana
physical sheath *see* annamaya kosha
PNS *see* parasympathetic nervous system (PNS)
polyvagal theory 144, 148, 149–53, 161; gunas and 162–3, **163**, 168
Porges, Stephen 144, 162
postures *see* asana postures
The Potter's Wheel metaphor 55
prakriti 50, 51–2, 87–8, *160*; constituents of 68–76, *69*, **70**, 78–9, 83–4; gunas and 57–66; metaphors for understanding 52–5; practices 56–7, 75–6
prana 95, 98–9, 104–8, 161
prana vayu meditations 98, 226–8, 243–5
prana vayus 95–8, **96**, *160*, 161, 171–2
pranamaya kosha 88–9, 89, 91–9, *91*, 114, 127–8, 129, 161
pranamaya reflection 221, 222, 224, 225
pranayama 15, 139, *160*, 170–2; for body-mind regulation 164, 204–7; for discriminative wisdom 223–6; for interoceptive and proprioceptive skills 223–6; for resilience and transformation 240–2; for sattva guna 164, 204–7
pranayama kosha meditation 223–6
pratyahara 174, 175, 206
proprioceptive skills: asana for 173, 217–23, 248; meditation practices for 220–9; pranayama for 223–6; yamas and niyamas for 214–17
psychological domain of health 114, 128, 129
psychophysiological perspectives 159–66, *160*, **163**
purusha 50–2, 87–8, *160*; gunas and 58, 62, 64; metaphors for understanding 52–5; practice 56–7

raga 81–3
raja guna 57–66; in body, mind, and environment 59–64, 72, 73, 75; definition 58–9; imbalanced 61–2; neural platforms and 162, 163, **163**, 165–6, 167–9, *168*; practice 65–6
reductionist approach 9, 124–5
regulation and resilience: asana for 164, 188–96, 191–3, 193–201, 236–40, 247–8, 249; meditation practices for 164, 207–11, 242–7; neurophysiological perspectives 137–42, 161; pranayama for 164, 204–7, 240–2; psychophysiological perspectives 162–6, **163**; yamas and niyamas for 183–8, *184*, 235–6; yoga therapy framework for 167–9, *168*; yogic perspectives 162–6, **163**; *see also* autonomic nervous system (ANS)
relaxation response 137, 138
resilience: asana for 236–40, 249; meditation practices for 242–7; neurophysiological perspectives 138–42, 161; pranayama for 240–2; psychophysiological perspectives 162–3, **163**, 165–6; types 232–5; yamas and niyamas for 235–6; yoga therapy framework for 167–9, *168*; yogic perspectives 162–3, **163**, 165–6
respiratory sinus arrhythmia 140–1, 150
right action 25, 32–6, 37, 38, 39–40, 42
rotator cuff tendonitis 127–8

safe immobilization neural platform 153, 162, 163, **163**
safe mobilization neural platform 152, 162, 163, **163**
salutogenesis 132–6, *133*; *see also* autonomic nervous system (ANS); regulation and resilience
samadhi 174
samana vayu 96–7, **96**, 172
samana vayu meditation 98, 243–4, 245
samkhya 49–66, 87–8, 100, 161; constituents of prakriti 68–76, *69*, **70**, 78–9, 83–4; definitions of purusha and prakriti 50–2; metaphors for understanding purusha and prakriti 52–5; practices 56–7, 65–6, 75–6; prakriti and gunas 57–66; relationship to yoga 49–50
Samkhya Karika 6, 37, 50, 51–5, 57, 68, 69, 72–3, 83, 84, 95
samskaras 79, 84
santosha 24, 185, 187
sattva guna 57–66; asana for 164, 188–96, 191–3, 193–201, 247–8; in body, mind, and environment 59–64, 70–1, **70**, 72, 73; buddhi and 70–1, **70**, 73, 78–9, 83–4; definition 58; importance of 61; meditation practices for 65–6, 164, 207–11; neural platforms and 162, 163–4, **163**, 167–9, *168*; pranayama for 164, 204–7; yamas and niyamas for 183–8, *184*

satya 185, 187
saucha 187
self-actualization 36, 118, 120, 121–2
self-regulation: asana for 164, 188–96, 191–3, 193–201, 247–8; meditation practices for 164, 207–11; neurophysiological perspectives 137–42, 161; pranayama for 164, 204–7; psychophysiological perspectives 162–4, **163**; yamas and niyamas for 183–8, *184*; yoga therapy framework for 167–9; yogic perspectives 162–4, **163**; *see also* autonomic nervous system (ANS)
sense capacities *see* buddhindriyas
sensory withdrawal 174, 175, 206
Singleton, Mark 172
SNS *see* sympathetic nervous system (SNS)
social domain of health 114–15, 116–17, 128, 129
social engagement system 150–1, 152, 153, 162, 163–4, **163**, 165, 167
social isolation 116–17, 128, 129
spiritual domain of health 115, 117, 128, 129, 161; eudaimonic well-being and 117–22, *118*, *119*
Stoler Miller, Barbara 79
story, teaching through 16
stress response 135–6, 137; *see also* sympathetic nervous system (SNS)
subliminal intentions 79, 84
subtle body 86–108; anandamaya kosha *89*, 90, 93–4, *93*, 114–15, 128, 129; annamaya kosha 88, *89*, 89, 91–2, *91*, 114, 127–8, 129; chakras 99, 101, 105, 106, 107; granthis 99, 101, 105, 106, 107; Khandava Forest story 86–7, 104–8; manomaya kosha *89*, 90, 91–2, *91*, 114, 128, 129; meditation practices 98, 101–4; nadis 98–9, 101; prana 95, 98–9, 104–8, 161; prana vayus 95–8, **96**, *160*, 161, 171–2; pranamaya kosha 88–9, *89*, 91–9, *91*, 114, 127–8, 129, 161; tantra 87–8, 99–104; vijnanamaya kosha *89*, 90, 93–4, *93*, 114–15, 128, 129
subtle elements 69, 74
subtle-body maps 98–9
sushumna 98–9
svadhyaya 101, 188, 215, 230–1, 235–6; asana for 217–23; meditation practices for 220–9; pranayama for 223–6
sympathetic nervous system (SNS) 92, 129, 136, 143, 146–7; definition 137; neural platforms 151, 152, **163**, *168*

Taittiriya Upanishad 22, 88–91, *89*
tama guna 57–66; in body, mind, and environment 59–64, 70–1, **70**, 72, 73, 75;
buddhi and 70–1, **70**, 73; definition 59; imbalanced 61–2; neural platforms and 162, 163, **163**, 165–6, 167–9, *168*; practice 65–6
tanmatras 69, 74
tantra 87–8, 99–104
tapas 39, 188, 235–6
Taylor, Matthew 176
top-down neurocognitive processes 138–9, 142
transcendental connectedness 115, 117–18, *118*, 120, 125, 164
truthfulness *see* satya

udana vayu **96**, 97, 172
udana vayu meditation 98, 244, 245
ujjayi breathing 205–6
unilateral-nostril breathing 206
Upanishads 5, 22–3, 25–6, 95, 170; Brihadaranyaka 23, 79–80; Katha 22, 25, 78; Mundaka 25–6; Taittiriya 22, 88–91, *89*

vagus nerve 143, 148–9; polyvagal theory 144, 148, 149–53, 161, 162–3, **163**, *168*; vagal control 140–1
vayu meditations 98, 226–8, 243–5
vayus 95–8, **96**, *160*, 161, 171–2
ventral vagal complex **163**, *168*
vijnanamaya kosha *89*, 90, 93–4, *93*, 114–15, 128, 129
vijnanamaya reflection 222, 223, 224, 225
virtues 120–1, 125; in action 39–40; dharma and 32–6, 37; engagement with life and 37–8; eudaimonic well-being and 36–7; personal expression of 34–6, 40–1
visualization practices 99, 139, 175, 176
vital sheath *see* pranamaya kosha
vyana vayu **96**, 97–8, 172
vyana vayu meditation 98, 244, 245

Wallis, Christopher 91, 95, 99
Wheeler, Amy 101
Wilcox, Julie 220, 247
window of tolerance 233–4, 237–8, 241–2
wisdom sheath *see* vijnanamaya kosha

yamas and niyamas 32–3, 37, 39, 115, 121, 138, *160*, 169–70; ahimsa 33, 185, 187; for body-mind regulation 183–8, *184*; for discriminative wisdom 214–17; golden mean 184–6, *184*; for interoceptive and proprioceptive skills 214–17; for resilience and transformation 235–6; santosha 24, 185, 187; for sattva guna 183–8, *184*; tapas 39, 188, 235–6
yoga nidra 175

Yoga Sutras of Patanjali 6, 49, 79, 80, 81, 100, 101, 161, 170, 172, 174, 235

yoga therapy framework 124–7, *126*, *160*; psychophysiological perspectives 159–66, *160*, **163**; for regulation and resilience 167–9, *168*; yogic perspectives 159–66, *160*, **163**; *see also* domains of health and well-being; neurophysiological perspectives

yogic perspectives 159–66, *160*, **163**

yogic sleep 175

Yudhisthira 17, 30–1, 34–5, 41, 61, 74, 75